Dr. Koyfman, **I was having a lot of pain all over my body.** I prayed and asked God for guidance on the path I should take to receive my healing. . . . I began a series of colonics and immediately started to feel better . . ."
—*H.P.*

"The most remarkable thing about Dr. Koyfman is his genuine desire to help. He really wants to help you get your health back, and then he really wants to help you maintain it. This is the thing that impressed me the most. . . ."
—*S.W.*

"I had difficulties with breathing, depression, bad sleeping, and muscle pain. When I started my treatment in Dr. Koyfman's office, my health became much better even from the first visit. . . ."
—*D.D.*

Find more testimonials between the chapter and near the end of the book.

Koyfman Whole Body Cleansing

Healing through Cleansing

Book 3: Improve Your Digestion

Stomach

Small Intestine

Liver

Lymph...

by Dr. Yakov Koyfman, N.D.

Practical Guide to a Healthy Lifestyle

Dedication

This little book is dedicated to the idea

That cleansing one's body of the toxins we take in
(from our food, water and air)
is an essential pathway to optimum health;

That natural techniques,
which are gentle and powerfully effective,
can and do remove the majority of these toxins;

and

That properly practicing
simple everyday cleansing procedures
is an important element
in one's overall detoxification program.

This book is one in a four-part series entitled:

Healing through Cleansing.

Book 1 is about the cleansing of the main excretory organs, the colon, kidneys, lungs and skin.

Book 2 tells how to cleanse the organs located in the head and neck region, the brain, thyroid gland, eyes, salivary glands, ears, nose and sinuses, throat, tongue, teeth and gums.

Book 3 deals with cleansing the abdominal organs, the stomach, small intestine, liver, blood vessels and blood, lymph, sexual organs, joints and spine.

Book 4 presents the main principles of a healthy diet with simple recipes for preparing living food dishes and safe cooking techniques which help to prepare freshly cooked foods without losing vital nutrients. Includes a weight loss program.

Each of these books contain testimonials both in the beginning and at the end of the book.

Preface

This book is published not as a substitute for, but rather as a supplement to, the care of your professional healthcare provider. More specifically, the procedures described in this book are designed to support the body's immune system through cleansing specific internal organs and systems down to the cellular level. In this way the body can be freed from the toxins it has picked up over the years, and its natural healing capacity strengthened. The information and techniques in this book are preventative in nature for the improvement of human health.

The information and the techniques described in this book are *not* designed to provide medical consultation or advice, diagnosis, prognosis, treatment procedures or prescription of remedies for any ailment or condition as those terms might be defined or construed by any federal, state or local law, rule, regulation or ordinance. Specifically, this book is not intended to engage in anything that legally would constitute the practice of medicine. The author of this book does not claim to treat any disease or provide any cure.

Instead, the information in this book is designed to create a better understanding of how the human body is capable of taking in and/or storing various chemicals, waste products and unwanted biologic organisms that are detrimental to human health. Further, this book is designed to discuss the impact these have on the human body, and how their partial or complete removal is beneficial to your health. Additionally, by increasing your awareness of these processes, this book hopes to create a greater self-awareness of personal health.

Because each person is unique, the author encourages each reader to pursue a daily self-care program tailored to his or her particular situation, based on that person's own best evaluation of the circumstances and in consultation with his or her professional healthcare provider.

Contents

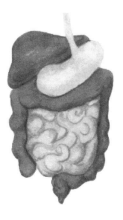

Introduction

In many ways our health depends on our lifestyle. Sometimes people who live an unhealthy lifestyle don't even know it because they don't understand what is a healthy lifestyle and what is an unhealthy lifestyle. Let's briefly describe these two ways of living.

An Unhealthy Lifestyle

An unhealthy lifestyle happens when you do not pay attention to your body and your health. People who live an unhealthy lifestyle assign either no time, or too little time, to improving their health. In addition, their diet and their lack of activity tends not toward improving health but toward destroying it. An unhealthy lifestyle pollutes and weakens the

1

whole system through the toxins it produces. Pollution to the system comes from poor diet, inactivity, poor blood and lymph circulation, lack of water and fresh air, wrong daily schedule, stresses and negative thinking, and also from the environment. Tiredness—being not just tired, but overtired, continuing to work or to work out when you feel tired, lack of rest and relaxation, and lack of sleep—is also related to an unhealthy lifestyle and increased pollution in the system.

A Healthy Lifestyle

A healthy lifestyle is the result of *the mind* having the knowledge it needs for good health, and *the will* having the wisdom and strength to implement that knowledge.

A healthy lifestyle is thinking, speaking, and acting in every way that leads to a **long life** *and* **high quality of living** without sacrificing any of the things in life that are truly enjoyable, profitable or natural.

A healthy lifestyle is **victory in living** not only for the physical body, but for the mind, the soul, and the spirit. As the body becomes healthier, so the mind thinks better and the soul and spirit become clearer.

A healthy lifestyle is **leaving behind the "pack mentality"** that is tragically symbolized by the lemmings that mythically race *en masse* over the proverbial cliff. It is not buying into *any* way of living that shortens your life or decreases the quality of living. It is not buying or using a product (or service) that is claimed to be good, but in reality is not. It is not allowing someone to treat your body with disrespect simply because he or she needs you to buy his or her product or service.

A healthy lifestyle is a **science** wherein the healing wisdom of the ages and the advantages of state-of-the-art medical science are blended together by both the experienced health professional and the informed patient.

A healthy lifestyle is an **art form** in which, once you have achieved your health goals through natural means, you walk through life exuding good health and leading others along the same victorious path.

A healthy lifestyle includes **cleansing your body** from toxins on all levels while faithfully maintaining that cleansing by following a rational diet.

Finally, a healthy lifestyle includes learning the necessary information about **proper exercise**, developing an exercise program tailored just for you, making time for that exercise program, and then actually doing the exercises on schedule.

People who live a healthy lifestyle constantly take care not just to cleanse the external body, but also to cleanse the internal organs. All of our organs and systems down to the cellular level require regular cleansing. Nature programs our bodies for this necessary maintenance to work automatically, but for many reasons our bodies become weak and cannot do this completely by themselves. They need help.

You—the individual in control of your body—are the first and most important element in achieving the optimum health possible for your body. Once you have decided to pursue this critical goal, you will need **reliable information**.

Our Center can recommend the following books to help guide you down the path of optimum health.

1. How to help clean your organs with professional help is described in my books: *Deep Internal Body Cleansing,* and *Eight Steps to Perfect Health.*

2. How to help your own system through self-help methods is described in my books, *Healing through Cleansing, Books 1-4,* and *Unique Method of Colon Rejuvenation.*

Abdominal Organs

The organs of the abdominal area include the stomach, small intestine, liver, gall bladder, pancreas, spleen, colon or large intestine.

The health of the digestive organs depends on a proper diet *and* on the cleanliness of those organs: the stomach, the large intestine and the small intestine. **Digestive organs are the most important channels of nourishing and cleansing the body.**

Where does the process of digestion start? In the stomach? No. In the mouth? Not always. Instead, digestion begins in the mind when you start thinking about food. If you are thinking about sweets, coffee or processed foods your digestion will be bad because the food is bad. This is because you will eat what you are thinking about. If you are thinking about a meal composed of fresh vegetables or fresh fruits, whole grains, breads, nuts, etc., your digestion will start off on the right foot: (1) choosing healthy foods and (2) the mind gearing up the rest of the body to receive good food. Never underestimate the power and influence of the mind to affect any part or function of the body.

The next step in the digestive process is in your mouth when you start eating. Two important elements of receiving nutrition begin in the mouth:

1. The start of the chemical breakdown of food.
2. The start of absorbing energy from food.

The very process of digestion releases energy contained in the molecules and the atoms of food. The energy of electrons is released when the food is chewed and by the chemical effect of saliva. Released energy is absorbed by the nerves of the mouth and spread through the whole body.

The mechanical breakdown of food by the teeth, and the chemical breakdown of food by saliva, prepare it for further digestion by the stomach and the small intestine. After these two organs are finished with the partially digested food, it goes to the colon for elimination. The cleanliness of these organs is important to their efficiency.

All the home cleansing methods described in this book are simple things you can do yourself for maintenance at any time. These methods *will not* completely cleanse your internal organs and systems from years-old toxicity. *Complete* cleansing can *only* be done in our Center under professional supervision.

To learn more about unique cleansing procedures done in our center, please visit our website at

w w w . k o y f m a n c e n t e r . c o m

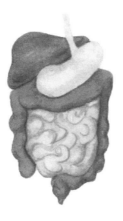

Stomach

As un-glamourous as this may sound, the stomach is a muscular "bag" in the shape of a pear. The inside surface of the stomach is covered by a mucus membrane which contains small glands that release stomach juices. The top right part of the stomach releases a very acidic juice, while the bottom left part of the stomach releases a less acidic juice. Toward the bottom of the stomach a "basic" digestive juice is released. In one day the stomach of an average person releases 1.5-2.5 liters (1.6-2.65 quarts) of stomach juice.

Although the entire human body is composed of innumerable chemical reactions, the stomach is the chemical laboratory where they all start. In the stomach food is sorted into nutrients and into waste. If the stomach receives food that has been properly chewed and sufficiently saturated with saliva, the stomach will operate like a well-oiled machine.

However if (1) the food that reaches the stomach has been gulped down without proper chewing, or (2) the food combinations are bad, or (3) the stomach is too full, or (4) the quality of food is poor, then the efficiency of the digestive process will suffer.

If any of this happens, instead of a healthy digestive processes that genuinely nourishes the body, you will get something unwanted such as fermentation or just plain decomposition. *(Just what you need: food rotting in your stomach, small intestine or large intestine.)* Unfortunately, this fermentation and decomposition can build momentum and become chronic. This situation can lead to such symptoms as headache, nausea, weakness, constipation or diarrhea. To make matters worse, an "impacted" stomach may send out hunger pangs at the wrong time, leading to bad eating habits.

In such cases it is necessary to cleanse the stomach. Fortunately the method of stomach cleansing is pretty simple. A description can be found in my book *Eight Steps to Perfect Health.* If you have decided to follow a healthy lifestyle you have to take measures to keep your stomach clean. And for your stomach to stay clean it is important for you to follow the right diet.

Aurvedic Tips on Diet

- Eat only when the stomach is ready for digestion; when you feel real hunger. This means that all food has left the stomach. Once this happens, the stomach has rested, filled up with juices and is ready for work.
- Sit up straight when eating.

- Stay away from conversations, reading or watching TV while you eat. Your attention should be focused on chewing properly and on the taste of the food.
- Most spices help to activate digestion and also improve the taste of food.
- Every piece of food should be chewed at least 32 times, and the more the better.
- Prolonged chewing helps to better physically break down food and saturate it with saliva for its absorption in the stomach.
- The amount of food consumed at one meal plays a big role in the quality of your digestion. An overfilled stomach stretches like a balloon. This has a negative effect on the heart and other organs. Too much food does not allow for a normal digestion. It stays in the stomach for too long and develops toxins.
- A good procedure to follow is to fill your stomach in the following manner: one third for food, one third for water that you drunk, and the last third will be for the digestive gasses which will be released.
- An individual portion for any person can be measured by however much food fits in both of his or her hands.
- Drinking lots of water during a meal is a bad idea. This is because people tend to let the water or other drink wash their food down before they have finished properly chewing. (The water permits larger sizes of food to go comfortably down the throat, whereas if water had not been drunk during the meal the person would have naturally chewed the food more to get it down.)
- Water or other drink consumed during a meal also interferes with the correct mixing of saliva with food. Saliva is meant to be the lubricant that gets food down our throats safely and comfortably. Since water or other drink has largely replaced

9

this function, food slips down the throat prematurely, and the chemical benefits of saliva as an initial digestive fluid are diminished.

- This is not to say that drinking small amounts of fluids from time to time while eating is a bad idea. This is because stomach juices are formed from water. That is why it is important to drink your water 15-20 minutes before any meal. Or if you wish, you can drink fresh fruit or vegetable juices 30-60 minutes before your meal.
- Additionally, if you drink a lot of water soon after eating, the water only dilutes your stomach juices and thereby inhibits proper digestion.

You can find other tips on how to improve the health of your stomach, how to properly combine foods, how to measure the best biorhythms for digestion, what to eat and what not to eat, in my book *Unique Methods of Colon Rejuvenation.*

Why We Need to Cleanse the Stomach

It has been said that, "As long as we live, breathe, eat and drink we are constantly polluting our bodies." Every time food moves through the stomach it leaves a trail. Incorrectly combined food, refined foods, sweets, dairy products, chemically contaminated food, eating late, overeating, eating on the run or under stress, not chewing enough, etc., all decrease the health of our digestive system, in particular the stomach.

I recommend that the average person do one stomach cleansing every month. You may learn under professional care how to cleanse your stomach. After 3-4 sessions, you may try to do it by yourself or continue to do it with professional help.

10

The benefit of professionally cleansing the stomach on this
schedule is that it activates digestive glands and the work of
the liver and pancreas, plus it removes toxins stored in the
stomach, sinuses, bronchi and lungs, but doing stomach
cleansing once a month is not enough. To keep your digestion
on a highly efficient level, you need to maintain its cleanliness
every day.

Everyday Methods of Stomach Cleansing

Method 1: Cleansing the Stomach after Each Meal

There is a great deal that the **average person can do on his
or her own without utilizing the services of a professional.**
These are actions that can be reasonably woven into the fabric
of everyday life so that digestion can deliver to you the
maximum nutrition your mind and body need.

**The first rule for stomach cleansing is not to eat again
until previous food is gone from the stomach.** Unless you
keep track of the time needed in the stomach for different
foods, the best way to determine this is the natural way.
Specifically, you experience a sensation of real hunger, not
some mere discomfort or stray feeling in the stomach. (See
discussion below.)

Be wary of the various tables and charts that purport to
provide reliable information on how long it takes to fully
digest a given food. Far too often, these tables are based on
their author's personal digestive system, and are not the result
of a true scientific study. These tables do not take into account
such factors as age, the health of the stomach, the health of the
rest of the digestive tract, or when the meal was eaten

11

(breakfast, dinner or supper). Because these conditions are not considered, one can find wide ranging differences for the same food in different tables. For example, the digestive time for meat is 2 hours in one table and 7-10 hours in another table. Some write that starch is digested in 2 hours, others give it 5 hours.

How can you tell the difference between real hunger and mere "discomfort"? "Discomfort" in the stomach is the result of worrying, anxiety, irritability, and a host of negative emotions, along with such physical conditions as bloating, light pain, or "the feeling that you need to eat something right away, but you don't want to cook, just grab something."

Real hunger does not cause irritability, weakness, etc. Instead you feel active and energetic, with a desire to cook something healthy and life-giving. Your stomach feels empty and light. Your mouth is moisturized with saliva.

Method 2: Morning Cleansing

This is a good time to drink a glass of water with 1-2 teaspoons of **organic apple cider vinegar,** or a glass of water with **freshly squeezed lemon juice.** These will have a cleansing and disinfecting effect on the walls of the stomach.

Another thing you can do for the health of your stomach is to drink tea made from bitter herbs such as **dandelion root tea** and others. This will help activate and cleanse the stomach, the pancreas, and the liver.

Method 3: Cleansing the Stomach If You Ever Get Nauseated

You can find relief from nausea by drinking water mixed with organic apple cider vinegar. (Yes, I know that sounds tough to do on a sick stomach, but this has been field tested extensively. What you want is something that works.) Add one teaspoon of apple vinegar to eight fluid ounces of water. Drink two little sips every five minutes until you drink 3-4 glasses of this beverage. Your stomach will be cleansed and nausea will pass.

Method 4: Aurvedic Methods of Stomach Cleansing

This method is good when you have toxins or indigestion.

Boil water for 10 minutes to destroy any bacteria that may possibly be in the water. (Yes, you should be using very pure water anyway, but this will make sure.) Pour this water into a thermos to retain the temperature throughout the day. Drink one or two sips every 5-10 minutes for three or four hours, or even for the whole day. Since this water is very hot, you may need to pour the sips into a glass at first to keep from burning your lips and mouth. You do want to avail yourself of the heat energy in the water. As an alternative you may wish to try adding one to two teaspoons of lemon juice to a glass of water.

Method 5: Cleansing of the Stomach Through Fasting

This method works both ways: for prevention, and for help with upset stomach, digestive problems, or other stomach disorders.

Water and Juice Fasting. For 24-36 hours do not eat anything. Instead, consider one or more of the following:
• Drink distilled water
• Drink freshly squeezed fruit juice or vegetable juices, strained to remove most solids.

13

Dry fasting. Dry fasting is more powerful as a stomach cleanser, but it requires more will power. Do not eat or drink anything for 8-24 hours. Afterwards *slowly* drink a glass of clean water, and *slowly* start eating. Fasting will not only cleanse the stomach but will also give it some rest, which will positively affect its work.

Method 6: Chlorophyll Cleansing

This method is helpful when you have irritation or burning.

Good stomach cleansers are the various green juices containing chlorophyll such as wheat grass juice, barley juice, and others. You can dilute them in a glass of water and drink them in the morning on an empty stomach. Chlorophyll is considered to be an internal deodorant.

Important Note: In serious cases, stomach cleansing must be done under professional care with vomiting techniques. See my book, *Eight Steps to Perfect Health.*

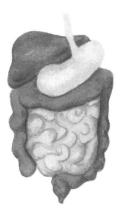

Small Intestine

After the stomach finishes working its chemical magic on the food you have eaten, this partially digested food is sent the second major chemical factory in the human body, the small intestine.

The small intestine is a tube-shaped organ 20-30 feet in length, depending on the size of the person. Its inside surface is covered by hair-like cells which control the movement of food through the small intestine. These hair-like cells also secrete intestinal juices while absorbing nutrients.

One of the "tools" used by the small intestine is a chemical called bile. Bile is manufactured by the liver, collected in the gall bladder and then secreted into the small intestine to help digestion. Bile neutralizes the effects of stomach juices, whose job has now ended. It also accelerates the effect of pancreatic juices during the breakdown of fats and prevents the decay or rotting of food in the small intestine. The amount of bile released by the liver during the day can reach up to one liter (about one quart).

Pancreatic juices are manufactured by the pancreas, which is located behind the stomach. Pancreatic juices work on fats so that they can be absorbed through the walls of the intestine. After the nutrients are absorbed and carried away by the blood, the remaining food is transferred to the large intestine, or colon. What happens here is discussed elsewhere, but suffice it to say that the very last nutrients are removed in the colon, and the waste is prepared for expulsion from the body.

Digestion and the Small Intestine

Too often the digestive system becomes a source of toxins, both chemical and biologic, which spread throughout the body. Emotional wastes (negative emotions) create constant tension in the small intestine, liver, and pancreas. But it's not only negative emotions that create tension in the muscles of the small intestine. Spending a long time in an uncomfortable position (especially the sitting position) also leads to the formation of blockages in these organs. As stated earlier, blockages lengthen the time it takes food to pass through the digestive system, and blockages also cause food to ferment and decay. This causes toxic substances and poisonous gasses to form.

Emotional duress or tension can lead to blockages in the small intestine. Additionally, gasses can block the small intestine. At this point, some people begin to wonder how something as "fluid" as a gas can block the tub-shaped passageway of the small intestine. Actually the explanation is simple. The small intestine causes material to move through it

by sequentially squeezing its ring-shaped muscles. If gas is present in large enough quantities, the gas can push against the walls of the small intestine enough to hinder its ability to squeeze. In this scenario, the small intestine simply can not function. This is essentially a blockage because material can not move forward. (This same process can and does happen in the colon.) Gas can form in the small intestine for a variety of reasons:
• Poorly chewed food.
• Improper food combining.
• Many healthy foods produce a large amount of gas (cabbage, broccoli, beans).
• Overeating.
• Eating late at night.
• Eating low quality food.

Methods of Small Intestine Cleansing

Colon Method

First make sure the large intestine is properly cleansed. The logic here is very simple. The small intestine pours its contents into the large intestine. If the large intestine is blocked by accumulated waste, then there is nowhere for the material in the small intestine to go. This makes it all the more likely that the small intestine will itself become clogged with material that should have been excreted. If the small intestine is not cleared out properly, its wastes can poison the liver and the pancreas. That is why it's important to maintain a clean colon, which would help in cleansing the small intestine, liver and pancreas.

Massage Methods

Massage is an effective method of preventing and removing blockages in the small intestine. (Look carefully at any graphic of the human digestive system to remind yourself where the main internal organs are located.) The small intestine is located at the center of the abdomen around the navel. Organs in the abdominal area are very close to the skin. If you press on your abdomen you can feel your stomach, small intestine, etc. Of course, if your abdomen is covered by a thick layer of fat it will be more difficult, but not impossible. (If you are reading this book it is obvious that you are taking your health seriously. If you follow the recommendations in this book, and my other books, you will soon loose that extra weight.)

Self-massage of the small intestine is best done in the morning after waking, while lying on your back. Also, you may do this before you go to sleep at night.

Self-massage of the small intestine is performed clockwise following the natural curves the small intestine makes in your abdominal cavity. Apply light pressure with your fingers or your palm, and go in circles starting with the navel and gradually moving outward. If you are massaging exposed skin it is better to moisten your fingers with some massage oil. But if you are massaging through the clothes your dry fingers will easily slide over them. If you perform this massage everyday you will soon learn to locate tensed and blocked areas. Give these areas a little extra attention until you can feel that each area has became softer.

Fruits Method

This method is based on eating in-season fruits for a whole day. The theory and practice of this method will be described in the chapter on lymph cleansing.

Note: Full cleansing of the small intestine must be done under professional care once every season, four times a year. See my book, *Eight Steps to Perfect Health.*

"Clean Feeling Inside"

During the colonic . . . I would say it was indescribable. It's something like limbo, you feel suspended. It is an exercise in relaxation. Afterward it's a payoff because you feel significantly better and nothing could duplicate the particular kind of clean feeling inside.

- Lucy Kern, 29 years old

"...Having a severe yeast overgrowth is not fun at all. Constant yeast infections, antibiotics from doctors, creams and other junk to treat it felt endless. Nothing ever helped and only made it worse. Only through Dr. Koyfman I found out that yeast is actually an intestinal diseases. During my first Small Intestine procedure I saw so much yeast come out, it was unbelievable. I kept my diet strict for a few days and felt amazing since than! No more gas, bloating, vaginal yeast, brain fog, fatigue. I cannot believe it was all do to that small parasite..."

Debbie K.

Dear Koyfman Staff,

For three years I have felt very sick. Horrible stomach pain, nausea and vomiting almost daily. After visiting this center for only three times I have felt a complete turnaround. My digestion is so much better. I am actually able to eat and not vomit afterwards. After my first Small Intestine Cleansing procedure something amazing happened. I came out from the center and realized that I don't have an urge to smoke. I didn't smoke since that moment.

I say complete "turn around" but know I will fill even better after all of my sessions are complete. Thanks to this clinic I can finally get on with my life. This clinic in fact saved my life. I can't thank you enough. Oh, and Dr. Koyfman, let me know if you ever decide to move anywhere, 'cause I'm going wherever you do!

Very Truly Yours,
Nick S., 26 years old

"I Have Never Felt Better in My Life!"

I think that the idea of body cleansing is the best thing that I've come across in a long time! I believe that every person on this earth can benefit from this. The Koyfman Whole Body Cleansing is one of the best offices I've ever been to. Dr. Koyfman is an extremely intelligent and experienced doctor! I have never felt better in my life!

- Catherine H., 29 years old

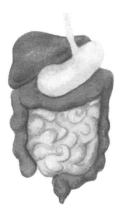

Other Internal Organs

Stomach, Liver, Gall Bladder, Spleen, Colon, and Reproductive Organs

The same benefits of self-massage as listed for the small intestine apply to other organs in the abdominal area: stomach, liver, gall bladder, spleen, and colon. Blockages caused by unexpelled wastes and gasses can be lessened or removed by the knowledgeable massage of these organs.

First, make sure you locate the organs you wish to massage on a chart of the human body so you know exactly where to find them on your own body. By massaging the entire

21

abdominal area you can lessen or remove blockages from these organs, and improve the circulation of blood and other fluids in these organs.

During your self-massage you do more than release tension, remove blockages and speed up the movement of food through digestive tract. You also cause gases to move, either up or down along the digestive tract. If gases move upward you might experience burping. This is normal during such a massage, and shows that energy is moving. This kind of self-massage is useful in the morning right after waking up, or during exercises, and it is also useful after a meal.

After each meal you may wish to go for a short walk during which you lightly massage your abdomen clockwise. Being in a vertical position during a walk decreases the amount of tension in the internal organs. A short walk combined with deep breathing energizes the body, gives more oxygen to the cells, improves the work of the heart, and generates the energy necessary to properly start digestion. Massaging the abdomen also stimulates circulation in the stomach, pancreas, liver and other organs while helping break down blockages and utilize available nutrients more efficiently.

If you choose to consciously help your internal organs every day in the work they must perform, you will decrease the amount of accumulated waste in those organs, and make it easier for your immune system to function optimally. The regular massage of the abdomen is a useful part of helping to rid your internal organs of waste, and helping each one to work more efficiently. This massage can improve the circulation and cleansing of all organs including the **kidneys, bladder and reproductive organs (uterus, ovaries, etc.).**

There are specific techniques for the proper massage of each internal organ. These specific techniques are based not only on the shape and location of the organ in question, but are also based on other characteristics of that organ. Although a great deal of valuable information can be learned from books, learning how to massage an individual internal organ is best done with a skilled professional, not from a book. (Several human endeavors fall into this category, sex being an indisputable example of a topic that is **not** best learned from books.) Training in internal organ massage techniques is taught at my Center.

A secondary, and adequate, means of learning internal organ massage is through video. Although video lacks the "feel" that is learned in private one-on-one training, it does show the motions that books can not show. Video is also a great reminder on "how-to" after being taught professionally. I am planning to produce just such a videotape in the future. For now, those who would like to learn these techniques are welcome to schedule a class at our Center to be instructed.

In the meantime, even if you have not received any professional-level training in internal organ massage, it would be better for you to just "wing it" and do the best you can on your own. This is because *something is better than nothing* as long as you do not press too hard and you do not have a medical problem in the area to be massaged. **Never** massage any injured part of your body, or an area that has had surgery without first consulting your health care provider. Remember, pain is nature's way of telling you something is wrong. Massage should feel good, or in the case of deep tissue massage, some small discomfort may be felt, but not pain.

Please remember that the benefits of every kind of massage are temporary since tensions and blockages too quickly reappear. That's why its important to regularly and professionally cleanse internal organs, and on a daily basis perform self-massage on your internal organs. The frequency of professional cleansing of internal organs is described in my book, *Eight Steps to Perfect Health.*

Exercises that Cleanse and Massage the Internal Organs

Certain yoga exercises are excellent for massaging internal organs. This is because yoga exercises were thoughtfully designed to move the body in very careful ways that stimulate the body beneficially. Exercises appropriate for this are described in my book, *Unique Method of Colon Rejuvenation,* specifically exercise number 4 - *The Rocking Chair*, exercise number 5 - *Reaching for the Earth* and exercise number 6 - *Reaching for the Stars*. These exercises improve circulation in the abdominal organs, and thereby supply them with energy. These exercises also strengthen and cleanse these organs.

Cleansing and Massaging Abdominal Organs by Breathing

As natural as breathing is, the average person living in an industrial nation does not breathe correctly. This is due to a wide variety of reasons: overeating that swells the stomach and presses against the diaphragm, our sedentary lifestyle with its lack of exercise that tend to atrophy the lungs, and the stomach being filled with gases and wastes that also press against the diaphragm. Whenever you press against an organ for a long time the pressure tends to impede that organ's circulation, waste removal and overall function. The diaphragm and the lungs are no exception.

After you have your colon, small intestine, liver and other internal organs professionally cleansed, these negative effects on the diaphragm and lungs will disappear. You will feel lighter, and your diaphragm will function more easily.

There is a way to "constantly" massage your internal organs to increase circulation, and by this prevent stagnant conditions from forming. It is called "Diaphragmatic Breathing," and is based on the fact that the diaphragm is under our conscious control. Fortunately it is easy to learn.

Diaphragmatic Breathing Technique

Lie on your back and relax. Put the palm of your right or left hand on the center of your abdomen. As you inhale slowly and deeply (not too deeply) move your hand upward with your abdomen, and as you exhale (slowly) move it downward. The purpose of using your hand in this fashion is to help emphasize the use of the diaphragm in breathing. Use your hands only while learning diaphragmatic breathing. When you have mastered this beginning technique lay your hands beside your body and relax. Now take slow, deep breaths using your diaphragm to breathe.

You can start with 10 of those breaths in the morning and another 10 breaths in the evening, gradually increasing to 15-20 times. If you perform this breathing for one to two months, your respiratory system will learn to breathe in this way all the time. This system of breathing will create a constant diaphragmatic massage and cleansing of the abdominal organs.

When lungs fill up with air during diaphragmatic breathing, the diaphragm moves downward pushing on the abdominal organs, stretching and massaging them. This movement activates circulation, peristalsis, removes blockages, etc. When we exhale, the diaphragm is moving upward pulling the abdominal organs with it. This action gently massages them.

Simple Exercise to Release Tension from the Abdominal Organs

There is another simple and easy exercise designed to cleanse your abdominal organs. It is one you can do in your office, or at home, while sitting in a chair or on the floor. In order to better understand the value of this exercise first realize that when people sit down they tend to compress their abdominal muscles. This is a result of leaning slightly forward and of curving the spine. This compression slows the circulation of these organs.

The technique for this exercise is to sit down in a natural position. Then reach your hands up in the air as if you were stretching, or signaling a touchdown in football. Simultaneously, arch your spine backward and look upward so that your abdominal cavity is "opened" as you lean (safely) backwards. The value of this exercise is that it gets rid of the cramped position the abdominal organs are usually in, relaxes them and decreases tension. This also increases circulation of the blood, lymph fluids, bile and other bodily fluids. Repeat this exercise about every one to two hours.

Mental Energy Massage of Internal Organs

Manipulation of Organs and Exercise of Vessels

Mental Energy Massage is a unique method through which we can control and make a difference in any organ or system of the body. With the help of this massage we can touch any part of the organism or any organ: muscles, stomach, liver, blood vessels, glands, spine, bones, joints, lymph, . . . everything.

I used this massage successfully for many years without even knowing that it was a Mental Energy Massage. The usual reaction of humans to pain is to try to get the mind off that part of the body or organ so as to forget and not feel the pain. I always did the opposite. I intentionally focused my mind into the depth of the pain, mentally trying to wash away the tension and ease the pain. It always brought good results.

The tool of the Mental Energy Massage is thought. With the help of thoughts we can enter deeper than hands or other tools could go. Thought is psychological energy capable of producing or changing the feelings in different organs. Thought which is activated by the imagination produces stronger feelings and quicker changes. With the help of thought in muscles and organs, we can bring up feelings of relaxation, warmth, tingling, cold, calmness, etc. The manifestations of these sensations can move in different ways: circle, straight line, zig-zag, back and forth. The manifestation of a healthy effect is the appearance of healing in that part of the body.

Healing in an organ or other part of the body is possible when the pathway of energy is complete from the brain to the organ. When you concentrate well enough so as to relax other tensions and to feel an organ, you have increased the connection of this organ with the brain and improved its function and control. When you start feeling the organ or its part, you expand the blood vessels in that area and improve circulation. Improving circulation delivers better nourishment and better cleansing to that organ. Mental Energy Massage eliminates the base of pain, tension, and spasm, which could be the cause of stress or blockages in different organs.

If the simple feeling of the organ or its part yields such positive effects to the system, then producing feelings of relaxation, warmth, tingles, or cold brings even more benefits because these feelings open even more blood vessels and further improve circulation. Alternating feelings of warmth and cold several times expands and shrinks the blood vessels, making them more flexible. This is Mental Blood Vessel Exercise and, in conjunction with cleansing diet and physical exercise, it helps to cleanse blood vessels and heal from many serious illnesses. To increase the effect of alternating feelings of warmth and cold, it is helpful to introduce tingling. Tingles intensify feelings of warmth and cold.

How to Do Mental Energy Massage

- Sit in a comfortable chair or lie on a bed or on the floor, and relax.
- Relax your face, especially your forehead. Relax your hands, legs, body, and especially your shoulders and breathing muscles. Calm your breathing, which leads to calming the whole system.
- Concentrate on the organ you want to improve, and feel it.
- Visualize your hand massaging that organ, squeeze and relax. Do this for 30-60 seconds.

- Move your thoughts through that organ in different directions, circles, zig-zag, straight line, back and forth, for 30-60 seconds.
- If you experience pain in some part, transform your thoughts into fire and burn it.
- If you know you have tumor in that organ, make your thoughts like a scalpel or laser and eliminate the tumor.
- Mentally grow the new healthy part and fill up what is missing in the organ.

How to Do Mental Blood Vessel Exercise

- Create feelings of warmth in the organ (visualize hot steam, hot water, sun) for 30 seconds. Turn the warmth to tingles for 30 seconds.
- Create feelings of cold (visualize ice, wind, snow, freezer) for 30 seconds, and finish with tingling from the cold for 30 seconds.
- Repeat this cycle three times: feelings of warmth then tingling, feelings of cold then tingling.
- Finish the work with each organ by using the following formula, stated convincingly. This is a sample statement to be adapted for each organ: "My liver is absolutely healthy, and I'm feeling good and strong."
- Take a break for a few minutes and, if you wish, work with another organ.

To reach the goal, do the Mental Energy Massage and Mental Blood Vessel Exercise 30-40 days for each organ you want to support. The best condition for success is regularity of performing the massage and exercise and belief in success.

With the Goal of Prevention and Healing, Work with These Organs

• Working with the spine activates energy centers, or chakras, improving the function and control of vital organs throughout the whole system.
• Working with any organ improves its function and healing.
• Working with glands improves their function and blood.
• Working with the blood vessel system improves circulation, strengthens the blood vessels and makes them more flexible, normalizes blood pressure, and helps with varicose veins and hemorrhoids. In conjunction with colon and liver cleansing, it helps to cleanse blood vessels.
• Working with bones improves the function of bone marrow, which helps to improve the immune system.

To learn more about unique cleansing procedures done in our center, please visit our website at
www.koyfmancenter.com

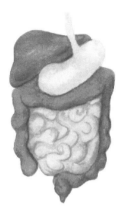

Liver

Every human being on this planet has toxins stored in his or her liver. The reason for this is simple: the liver is designed to filter the blood of impurities such as toxins. Dr. Schulz said about the liver, **"Your liver is your first line of defense and your body's main detoxifying organ. For most people it's a toxic garbage dump overflowing with waste and poisons."**

The liver is a chemical factory for the body; it's a fuel storage warehouse, and it is your "poison control center." The work of the liver directly affects the proper function of the kidneys, spleen, heart and other organs. If the liver is not functioning well and doesn't filter blood properly, the channels of endocrine glands, which are very narrow, become clogged and start to dysfunction. This is especially true for the thyroid gland.

The liver is the largest gland in the human body weighing up to four pounds. On average the liver filters 1.5 L (about 1.5 quarts) of blood per minute. The entire volume of blood in the body passes through the liver in 4-5 minutes.

Venous Stagnation

Lack of proper diaphragmatic breathing can result in venous stagnation. ("Venous" refers to the veins as opposed to the arteries.) Stagnation of blood in the veins can, in turn, lead to spider veins, poor liver function, constipation, diseases of the thyroid gland, and even cancer of the breast and reproductive organs. In fact, venous stagnation opens the gates to all sorts of infections and diseases.

Methods of Combating Venous Stagnation and Cleansing the Liver

There are at least four different things that can be done to prevent the stagnation of blood in the veins. These are:
• Learning "Diaphragmatic Breathing," described in the previous chapter.
• Removing the pressure of abdominal organs on the diaphragm. This is achieved through regular cleansing and proper diet.
• Massage and self-massage of internal organs. It is better to do self-massage of internal organs of the abdomen while laying on the slanted board. (See information on a slant board in the back of this book.)
• Warm bath or heating pad also decreases venous stagnation in the liver and other organs.

Liver Cleansing: *Heat Method*

If you take a warm bath for 15-20 minutes, or put a heating pad on your liver for 30-60 minutes, you will warm up your liver and your blood by a few degrees. Warming up your blood even by one degree increases its ability to kill microbes by 10 times. The Far Infrared Ray (FIR) machine is especially good at deep heating the liver and widening its channels which helps its natural cleansing. An FIR machine is often used in my center. A warm bath also helps in widening the channels of the liver and removing toxins from liver and bladder.

Anatoli Malovichenko says that **"without cleansing and regular heating of the liver you can't cure any serious disease."**

The typical modern American diet makes blood more acidic, which in turn leads to the formation of "aggressive toxic bile." Aggressive toxic bile has the nasty habit of irritating the bile channels. Additionally, if you eat late in the day, particularly less than four hours before going to sleep, late night digestion and an overfilled stomach can put pressure on the liver, making its work harder. Being in a horizontal position during sleep, and that pressure from the stomach, can transfer aggressive toxic bile to the pancreas where it can do damage. If the pancreas is in a weakened state, eating sweets can more easily lead diabetes. An overfilled stomach at night also inhibits the flow of bile into the small intestine. Bile accumulates in the gall bladder, gets pressed together and forms gall stones.

Just as the kidneys and the gall bladder can form "stones," so also can the liver. Liver stones are composed of toxic substances filtered from the blood. During a liver cleanse, hundreds of these stones can be released. When these stones stay in the liver and gall bladder they can cause problems.

In the small intestine, aggressive toxic bile cannot completely break down fats. Instead, what you get is a mixture of fats and this bile absorbed into the blood stream. This sometimes causes allergic reactions and skin problems. The circulation of blood in the liver strongly depends on the movement of the diaphragm.

Liver Cleansing: *Diaphragm Method*

The diaphragm is a very powerful muscle that expands and contracts in order to work the lungs so that we can breathe. As it expands, the lungs are compressed and we exhale. When the diaphragm contracts, the lungs expand and we inhale. If the colon is not full of stored wastes, and does not interfere with the movement of diaphragm, it makes about 18 cycles per minute. This means 1000 cycles per hour and 24,000 in a day.

When the diaphragm expands it squeezes not only the lungs, but the liver, spleen and other abdominal organs as well. This stimulates the circulation of all fluids in the abdomen. Good circulation leads to better cleansing and better delivery of nutrients to all of these organs. By putting pressure on all blood and lymph vessels of the abdomen, the diaphragm pushes the blood and lymph towards the chest cavity. This greatly helps the heart by preventing accumulation of blood in the abdomen. This is why the diaphragm is often called the second heart.

Liver Cleansing: *Juice Methods*

On a more nutritious note, a wonderful agent for liver cleansing is beet juice. Beets contain 50 percent sodium, 20 percent potassium, 8 percent chloride and 5 percent calcium. These proportions help cleanse the liver, bladder and kidneys, plus dissolve calcium in blood vessels. Beet juice is also beneficial for problems with veins, hypertension and heart disease.

This juice can be consumed by itself, or in combination with different vegetables and fruits. Because it is particularly powerful in cleansing the liver, people who have never consumed beet juice should dilute it with carrot or apple juice. Then as they see how it affects their liver, digestive system and excretory system, they can drink beet juice that is less dilute. Newcomers to beet juice should remember that it colors both urine and feces a beet-like color. So don't be too shocked when you see that your urine has turned a shade of burgundy.

Some Recipes for Beet Juice in Combination with Other Juices

- Carrots (5 ounces) and Beets (3 ounces).
- Granny Smith Apples (12 ounces) and Beets (4 ounces).

Daily consumption of one to two (1-2) glasses of the above combinations of juices will ensure regular cleansing of the liver if done in combination with the following:
- The liver has been professionally cleaned, recently and thoroughly.
- The liver is not abused by a rotten diet that clogs it up again.

35

- Other recommendations on liver health found in this book are followed.

Remember that the liver is the most important filter in your body, and is the most important organ you have for fighting cancer. If you keep this filter clean using the techniques described in this book, you can be sure that your liver will be able to do its part in defending your body against the innumerable bacteria and viruses that assault each of us almost daily.

Foods, Herbs and Other Products Which Enhance Liver Cleansing

- Beets.
- Carrots.
- Apples.
- Black radish.
- Dandelion root tea.
- Olive oil.
- Honey.

Try to include these in your diet.

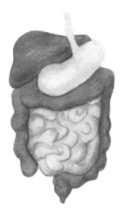

Blood Vessels and Blood

Problems with Arteries, Veins, Capillaries, and Blood

If you have ever seen plumbing pipes clogged with grease, you have a good idea what it is like in the veins and arteries of the average, modern American eating the sticky processed food so typically eaten in this country.

Stagnant blood, loaded with artificial chemicals, fats, excess cholesterol, and various wastes, deposits one thin layer of plaque after another onto the walls of our veins and arteries. Over time, these deposits build up thickly enough to restrict blood flow and thereby increase blood pressure. It is this situation that too often ends up in coronary arrest and death.

Some people think that they are safe from cardiovascular disease until they are middle aged or older. Nothing could be further from the truth. Autopsies performed on soldiers who were killed in Vietnam showed conclusively that the standard American diet had already begun to deposit significant amounts of plaque on their arterial walls. So just because noticeable symptoms do not show up until later in life does not mean the problem started then. It starts much earlier; for some people cardiovascular disease begins in childhood.

There is also the problem of elasticity in the blood vessels. A lack of vitamin C is considered by many health professionals as leading to veins and arteries being less elastic. In this case, the walls of the blood vessels develop miniature cracks that threaten to break through if not repaired. These health professionals believe that the body responds by filling these cracks with cholesterol or plaque. As time goes on, the process continues, and the veins and arteries begin to clog. This, of course, brings us again to the importance of eating good foods, and avoiding bad foods.

Most health problems are connected to disruptions in healthy blood circulation like those described above. During such disruptions, blood cannot deliver all the necessary oxygen and nutrients to the cells of the body. It is also unable to efficiently remove waste products generated when cells "burn" the nutrients they do receive. This results in those parts of the body being poisoned by wastes that linger. These two conditions, deficit of nutrients and increased toxicity, weaken the body's defenses, and are a prime reason for disease.

Non-organic foods, particularly processed foods, eating late, overeating, etc. are typical reasons for (1) toxins being formed in our bodies, (2) blood vessels being clogged and (3) circulation being disrupted.

"Least Wanted"

Some foods are notorious for causing excess mucus to form in the body. The leading villains here are no surprise: dairy products such as milk and cheese, white flour products, and refined grains. The problem with excess mucus is that it is not confined to the respiratory system and nasal passages. Indeed, mucus can be formed in virtually any part of the body, particularly in the colon.

Excess mucus creates several real health problems, such as making the work of the heart more difficult and providing an environment favorable for the formation of cancer. Proper professional cleansing of the colon and other organs, along with a proper diet go a long way towards ridding the body of excess mucus. People with sinus problems will experience some degree of relief, usually a great deal of relief.

Excess salt and fat are also bad for the circulatory system. Salt can and will accumulate on the walls of blood vessels making them hard and easily breakable. Excess animal fats turn into cholesterol which settles down in the liver and the walls of vessels making them more narrow.

Proper circulation of blood and other fluids can be inhibited by internal organs being swollen with accumulated waste. Such organs increase in size over time, and press against each other. Veins feeding blood to these compressed organs are also constricted leading to the circulatory problems discussed above.

By now you have probably anticipated another famous problem that seems to affect so many Americans today. That problem is our **sedentary lifestyle**. While we sit comfortably at home or at work, sometimes scarcely moving, the circulation of blood and other fluids slows down. It is at this time that a well-known law of sedimentology kicks in. When velocity in a fluid decreases, whatever it is carrying (sand in a river or contaminants in the blood stream) begins to fall out. In our context, artificial chemicals, fats, excess cholesterol, and various wastes tend to settle out and stick to the walls of veins and arteries.

Finally, **stress** is a factor to be considered in circulatory problems. Stress affects the nerves, which in turn create tension in muscles, organs and vessels. We have all seen people who are so uptight about one thing or another that even their muscles became hard and tense. So it should be no surprise that tension inhibits blood and other fluid flow within the human body.

Also during stress, certain hormones and other substances like glucose and fatty acids, are released into the bloodstream. These naturally-occurring substances are meant to be used by the body when it is under duress (fight or flight response to stress). In today's modern society that is allegedly not very frequent, but anyone who has driven in a high-speed rush hour in a big city can easily attest otherwise. Nonetheless, if stress causes your body to release these chemicals, the body wants to burn them. If this does not happen, then glucose and fatty acids will settle as fat on the walls of the vessels.

What Diseases Can Result from Impacted Vessels?

Hypertension

Hypertension is an increase in blood pressure on the walls of blood vessels. If one disregards age, normal blood pressure is 120/80. If blood pressure goes over 140/90 it is considered elevated. Sometimes blood pressure can get as high as 220/120 and more. Such increased blood pressure can be very dangerous, especially for vessels going through the brain, the heart and the kidneys. Signs of increased pressure can be frequent headaches, dizziness, decrease in work capability, fatigue for no apparent reason, problem sleeping, rapid heartbeat, and the feeling of pressure in the area of the heart. Under these conditions arteriosclerosis can develop (see below).

Low Blood Pressure

Low blood pressure is a decrease in the arterial blood pressure below 120/80. This condition most often effects young women. Signs of low pressure are dizziness, labored breathing, low exercise tolerance, chest pains. Signs of hypertension and low blood pressure are very similar. But with lowered pressure the skin becomes pale; and with increased pressure the skin is red, especially on the face. In the event of a sudden, big drop in blood pressure (below 80/40) the situation can rapidly become dangerous.

Arteriosclerosis

Arteriosclerosis occurs when plaque and cholesterol accumulate on the walls of arteries, veins, and capillaries. This accumulation builds up over the years, and slowly decreases the diameter of the passageway in the blood vessels. As this happens, blood flow is restricted and blood pressure is increased. In time, this passageway can become so narrow that it will completely close off the flow of blood.

Associated with this condition is the likelihood that the tissues of the blood vessels will become less elastic, and more susceptible to developing tears or cracks. When this happens along with increased pressure, it is possible for these vessels to break, spilling their blood into nearby tissues and denying blood to other starving tissues.

Reasons for the development of arteriosclerosis include improper eating, sedentary lifestyle, stress, and smoking. Arteriosclerosis can also be passed on genetically. If your parents or relatives have this problem the chances are greater that you will develop it also. Because the frequency of death from arteriosclerosis has increased by 100 times, and because this problem is now effecting younger people, even as young as 25 years old, it is especially important to do preventive cleansing and to lead a healthy life style.

We have described a number of diseases connected with plaque in blood and vessels. In addition to these, impacted vessels are a simptom of problems with the whole system: colon, liver, kidneys, and other organs. Therefore, problems with the vessels can lead not only to cardiovascular diseases but also to other diseases. **Vessels are the transport channels of our body through which nutrients are delivered to organs and cells and through which waste products are removed. If the vessels are blocked in some areas of the body then these areas do not get enough nutrients and have excess toxicity.**

This is a sure way of developing disease in those organs. Under these conditions, hypertension, low blood pressure, or arteriosclerosis can develop. Hypertension, low blood pressure, and arteriosclerosis can lead to cardiovascular problems, heart attack, stroke, and kidney failure.

Methods of Cleansing the Blood Vessels at Home

Diet

Principles of healthy eating are described in my book, *Deep Internal Body Cleansing*. Read the chapter entitled, "Diet for Rational Health." The main goal of diet in vessel cleansing is to keep from adding to the build-up on the walls of the vessels. It is recommended to consume garlic everyday, as garlic is a very effective vessel cleanser.

Juice

It is also a good idea to consume vegetable juices mixed with green salads. They thoroughly cleanse vessels and blood. Some examples follow:
• Carrots + 4-5 leaves of kale + 1 clove of garlic.
• Carrots + 2-3 ounces of beets + 4-5 leaves of romaine lettuce + 1 clove of garlic.
• Apples (3) + 4-5 celery sticks + 1 clove of garlic.

Another thing that is very good for removing cholesterol is **citrus juice.** Try this experiment: put some oil on your fingers and then try to wash it away with water. Notice that the oil does not wash off. Now put some lemon or grapefruit juice on your fingers and you will be amazed at how quickly you'll be able to wash the oil off. You can eat one lemon a day. If it's organic, you may eat it with the skin. Eat this lemon before eating a high protein meal. The acid will help with digestion and will cleanse the vessels once it has been absorbed into the bloodstream. Also, in the morning you **can drink a juice made from two oranges and one grapefruit.** Peel the oranges and grapefruit with a knife so the white layer remains intact and put them through a juice maker like a "Champion" juicer. The white part of the skin contains a large amount of minerals and vitamins. Also, the bitter taste stimulates the release of stomach and pancreatic juices. When these are absorbed into the bloodstream they aid with cleansing the blood and blood vessels.

Other combinations of citrus juices include:
• Oranges (3) + 1 lemon.
• Oranges (2-3) + 1 grapefruit + ½ lemon.
• Lemon (1) + 2 tsp. honey + 2 c. pure or distilled water.

Water

The quantity and quality of water that you drink is very important for vessel cleansing. You can find out about the individual daily portions of water in my book, *Unique Method of Colon Rejuvenation.* Water can be distilled or filtered, although distilled water works better for body cleansing. The quality of water is also important when cooking soups and grains. If you drink clean water at home but then go to a restaurant and eat food prepared with regular tap water, you might be doing more harm than good for your vessels. Of course, we can't completely eliminate all negative effects of environment and society, but if our efforts to stay healthy outweigh the negative input from the environment, we will be healthy.

Warm Baths

Warm baths with the addition of salts, herbs, lemon juice, vodka and ginger root dilate the blood vessels and activate blood circulation. This procedure, repeated twice a week on a regular basis, will aid in cleansing the vessels and capillaries. Examples of helpful bath additives follow:
• Add 2-4 c. sea salt, rock salt, or Epsom salt.
• Add ½ c. lemon juice and 1/4 c. apple vinegar.
• Add ½ c. vodka and ½ c. lemon juice.
• Add 1/4 c. ginger root or juice of black radish.

Stay in the bath for 15-20 minutes. If the bath is not too hot and you have good tolerance, you can stay in it for up to 30 minutes. Get out of the bath slowly after rinsing your face and neck with cool water. Then take a cool shower to close your pores and to give yourself an energy boost.

Contrast Shower

I have already discussed in Book 1 the usefulness of contrast shower in vessel cleansing. Multiple changes in temperature repeatedly dilate and constrict the vessels, cleansing them and making them more elastic. The contrast shower technique is described in Book 1, in the chapter on skin cleansing, the section entitled, "Blood Vessel Cleansing in the Shower."

Self-Massage

The skin contains many nerve endings which connect it to all of the organs and vessels. Because of these multiple nerve endings, massage is very effective to activate blood circulation not only in the skin, but also in muscles, organs, and all vessels and capillaries. All types of self-massage are helpful, but massage with a dry brush is the most highly recommended because it also opens up the pores of the skin, aiding its cleansing and improving its breathing.

Breathing Exercises

Breathing exercise, number 6 from the book, *Unique Method of Colon Rejuvenation,* helps to make vessels cleaner and more elastic. Short and frequent breathing makes vessels constrict whereas slow, deep breathing makes them dilate. For this reason, alternation between fast-short and slow-deep breathing has a positive effect toward strengthening the blood vessels.

Fasting

Fasting on water or on fresh strained juices for 24-36 hours does a great job of diluting toxins in the vessels and cleansing the blood. This kind of fasting is recommended once a week or once every other week.

If, during one of these fasts, you cleanse your colon with colon hydrotherapy, very few nutrients will remain in your digestive system. Your body will have to get nutrients from the next available source, the blood and blood vessels. In its first search for nutrients, it will take the worst part, the toxins, plaque, and cholesterol from the walls of the blood vessels. In this case the effect of the fast will increase dramatically.

Juices used during the fast to cleanse your blood vessels could be a combination of citrus juices or green juices like spinach, romaine lettuce, parsley, garlic, and carob. See recipes for green juices in Book 4 and in my book, *Eight Steps to Perfect Health.*

Your fasting can result in an even larger effect on blood vessel cleansing if you start your fast right after a small intestine cleansing, causing your digestive system to remain completely cleansed and empty. In this situation, blood and blood vessel cleansing happens much faster and is more effective.

If you prolong your fast up to 3-5 days, your vessels will become as healthy as those of an eighteen-year-old. Read about small intestine cleansing in my other books, *Deep Internal Body Cleansing* and *Eight Steps to Perfect Health.*

Exercises

Running, walking, working in the garden, and other kinds of physical activity stimulate the work of the heart, increase the number of working vessels and capillaries, and aid in blood vessel cleansing by the sheer speed of blood flow. The importance of physical exercises in achieving and maintaining good health is imperative. **If you can't find time to exercise then, according to the great yoga master, Svali Shivananda, you should not take time to eat either.** If you do find time to eat you should also be able to find time for exercise. **If you do your exercises regularly, you will start developing "exercise hunger"** the same way you feel hungry for food. This is actually a real hunger felt by all muscles, organs, and cells for activity. This hunger is caused by the fact that the delivery of nutrients to the cells is the most complete during physical activity.

Relaxation

Stress affects not only the muscles and organs but also the blood vessels. Stress contracts and tightens the blood vessels, increasing the pressure in the blood vessels and interrupting the feeding and cleansing of cells. This causes the accumulation of wastes in blood vessels and organs so that in some parts of the body we may start feeling discomfort and pain. The pain attracts our attention to this part of the body, and we try to listen to what is there. We start thinking negatively about this part of the body. Everything bad we know of or have heard happened to others we try to find in our own system. Even though the problem is not so bad, our negative thoughts create destructive programming and begin to destroy the good programming. In addition, fear tightens the blood vessels even more and increases the depth of the problem.

Conscious relaxation and positive thinking act in an opposite way. Focusing our attention on relaxing some parts of the body and organs with positive thinking absorbs our attention and releases tension from the blood vessels, thereby relaxing and expanding them.

Short Description of Technique. Lie on your back or sit in a comfortable chair. Try to find such a position for your hands, feet, legs, and head that the position itself promotes muscle relaxation. Inhale and exhale deeply and close your eyes. Say silently to yourself, "I am now relaxing and becoming calm." Repeat this phrase several times.

During this time try to imagine and feel relaxation in all the muscles in your body. Then pay attention to that part of the body which is bothering you. Try to visualize and feel everything you think.

Say in your mind, "All large blood vessels, all medium blood vessels, and all very small blood vessels are completely open and expanded over their whole length. Clean and healthy blood is completely cleansing the blood vessels. My blood vessels are becoming clean, expanded, and relaxed. I feel calm, healthy, and strong." Repeat these phrases several times until you start to feel comfortable, relaxed, and very calm.

Remember, thoughts program our lives. Learn to think positively.

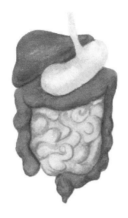

Lymph

Cleansing the Lymphatic System, Vessels, Blood and Tissue Fluids, and Cleansing from Heavy Metals

The lymphatic system is the body's means of collecting tissue fluids from intercellular spaces. The lymphatic system consists of lymph vessels and lymph nodes. The vessels start from intercellular spaces as very small lymphatic capillaries. Then the capillaries flow into larger lymphatic vessels. All of the lymphatic vessels flow into two major ducts, which in turn flow into veins. By this means, the lymphatic system empties into the venous blood flow. Lymphatic vessels have a number of valves preventing the back flow of lymphatic fluid.

Lymphatic vessels are interspersed with lymph nodes. Lymph nodes are small formations of ball or oval shape. They are considered organs of blood formation and defense. Lymphocytes are formed in the lymph nodes. When lymphatic fluid flows through a lymph node, it is filtered from microbes from skin tissues, bacteria from intestinal tract, coal and other fine particles from bronchi, etc., all of which are destroyed by lymphocytes.

Major Functions of the Lymphatic System

- Maintenance of consistency in content and volume of tissue fluids.
- Return of protein from intercellular spaces to the blood flow.
- Participation in distribution of fluids in the body.
- Maintenance of the connection between tissues and organs, and between the lymphatic system and the blood.
- Absorption and transport of products of food metabolism, especially the transport of fats from the gastrointestinal tract into the blood.
- Providing a defense mechanism against disease and damage from pollution.

Lymph consists of lymphoplasma, lymphocytes and thrombocytes. There are no erythrocytes in the lymph of a healthy person.

Let me point out once again that the lymph nodes play the role of filters. If a body is filled with toxicity, and the colon and liver are impacted, then the lymph nodes get "clogged" faster than they can clean themselves. They accumulate disease-causing bacteria and various toxins from the intestines, bronchi, skin, etc. When the lymph nodes are "clogged" in such a way, they can no longer prevent the spread of toxins and bacteria.

The lymph nodes can become inflamed and toxins begin to move through the lymphatic system and spread throughout the whole body. *Instead of providing defense from infection and toxins, the lymphatic system becomes their distributor.* This is why it is so important to maintain the cleanliness of your body, and especially of the lymphatic system. **Having a clean lymphatic system is having a strong immune system.**

In our center, we devote a lot of attention to cleansing and renewing lymphatic system. After this cleansing you will experience an improvement in digestion and in the work of the liver, pancreas, kidneys, urinary tract, and joints. You will experience decrease or elimination of back joint pain, cleaner skin, cleaner blood vessels, stronger immune system, and increase in the body's ability to fight off disease.

The procedure of lymph cleansing in our center takes three days. Every morning, on an empty stomach, the client drinks a concentrated mixture of minerals, which acts like a magnet, drawing the old lymphatic fluid toward the digestive tract and kidneys through which it can be eliminated from the body with the feces and urine. New lymphatic fluid is formed from the combination of fresh juices, which the patient drinks 1 glass every 20-30 minutes for 6-8 hours.

- For those who have a less acidic stomach juice, we recommend a combination of citrus juices: lemon, orange and grapefruit.
- Those who have a more acidic stomach juice should stick with carrot and celery juices.

51

Then we use two machines. The first machine, GX-99, is used to drain lymph from the whole body through a specifically selected frequency of vibrations. This helps to move stagnant lymphatic fluid through the lymph vessels and nodes. Then with the help of the second machine, Lustre 98, we do the actual cleansing of the lymph nodes. The use of these machines is described in my book, *Eight Steps to Perfect Health,* in the instructions for lymph cleansing, section entitled, "Services Provided at the Center."

After that we include a procedure for cleansing the colon where some of the old lymph can still remain. This is followed by an infrared sauna, where old lymph is excreted through skin. Then we recommend a special diet, which should be followed for at least three days after this procedure.

A less sophisticated procedure of lymph cleansing can be done by you at home.

Lymph Cleansing at Home

Lymph cleansing at home was described by a Russian doctor Shadilov. During fruit season, once a week, in the morning on an empty stomach eat a small amount of greens consisting of parsley, dill, green onion, lettuce, etc. The main ingredient should be parsley. The rest of the greens increase the cleansing effect of parsley and improve the taste of this green combination.

Half an hour later you can start eating juicy fruits, which are in season. These could be plums, peaches, apples, oranges, grapefruits, melons, watermelon, or any other fruits or berries.

Eat the chosen fruits throughout the day.

What Is the Concept Behind this Procedure?

You eat parsley at the very beginning of this procedure. Parsley has disinfecting and antiseptic qualities. It contains large amounts of anti-oxidants: vitamin C, carotene, folic acid (vitamin B 9), etc. The most important thing is that parsley is a great diuretic. Parsley in the system stimulates the work of the kidneys. During an active urine production the rest of the fluids in the body are also moving more actively: blood, lymph and tissue fluids. As a result, the body excretes a lot of fluids which were stagnant for long periods of time. **This eliminates edema, and improves the work of the heart and of the entire cardiovascular system.**

Through eating fresh juicy fruit the old fluids which were excreted are replaced with fresh, live fruit juices, which have anti-oxidative, disinfecting and anti-acidic effects. **Therefore, all fluids of the body, blood, lymph and tissue fluids, are cleansed.**

One More Valuable Quality of Fruit Cleansings

In extreme situations, under excessive stress, an oxygen deficit, or hypoxia, can develop. It can also happen as a result of such diseases as bronchial asthma, diabetes, nerve diseases, etc. Not only stress and disease are responsible for the development of hypoxia. As a person ages his metabolic processes slow down and cellular bio-energetic potential decreases, which can result in hypoxia.

What Are the Symptoms of Hypoxia?

- Agitation of the nervous system.
- Increased frequency of breaths.
- Increased heart rate.
- Accumulation of under-oxidized products of metabolism.
- Disruption of acid-base balance, toward increased acidity, in the internal environment, blood, lymph and tissue fluids.

Fruits and vegetables contain substances which prevent and decrease the effects of hypoxia. These substances are called anti-hypoxicants. Here is a list of products containing anti-hypoxicants: raspberry, strawberry, blueberry, carrots, beets, cabbage, dill, garlic, and tomatoes. This list contains not only fruits but also some vegetables which can be used in lymph cleansing.

Seasonal lymph cleansings also cleanse the entire body. They are helpful for people of any age, especially for older people.

Practical Hints on Conducting Lymph Cleansing

1. All fruits and vegetables used in cleansing should be ecologically clean, that is, organically grown. If you can't follow that rule for all, then at least the greens should be organically grown. All products should be carefully washed and dried and fruits should be peeled. This will reduce the number of harmful chemical substances entering your body. We have already discussed that there are no more absolutely clean products on this earth.

2. The movement of lymph through your body is not achieved through heart contractions, but through contractions of the muscles of your body including the diaphragm. Therefore, to remove stagnant lymph, which becomes that way because of many tensions in muscles and organs, it is important to start moving the lymph. You have to make it circulate and flow throughout the body.

   a. This can be done only through physical activity: running, walking, exercising, or other physical labor in your garden or at home. It is always better to engage in physical activity outside. Recall the importance of oxygen in breaking down toxins. Physical activity pushes old lymph toward the channels of exit: colon, kidneys, skin and a little bit through the lungs and breathing. Because the body contains hundreds of stress blockages, the longer your physical activity continues the more old lymph you will eliminate. It is not practical to be superactive all day long, and everything, even exercise, should be done in moderation.

   b. Alternate different types of physical activity to work different groups of muscles. You can use mini trampoline.

   c. You can use passive activity with the Chi machine. Although your muscles do not participate in this exercise, all of the body fluids are actively flowing, including the lymphatic fluid. I remind you once again, physical activity is an important component of lymph cleansing.

3. It is very beneficial to get a sauna and also full body massage the day of the cleansing. This activates the flow of lymph through all parts of the body and improves the excretion of lymph through the skin and kidneys.

4. The daily amount of water needed is calculated by using the formula, your weight (in lbs.) divided by two gives the number of ounces of fluids necessary for one day. Fruits that you eat throughout the day on average contain 90% water. Therefore, you need to eat 15-29% more weight in fruit to get the right amount of ecologically clean water from the fruit. You may slightly increase the amount of water to increase urine production.
    Example: If you weigh 130 lbs., you need 130 divided by 2 equals 65 oz. of water. At 16 oz. per 1 lb., 65 oz. is approximately 4 lbs. Out of 4 lbs. of fruit you will get only 48 oz. of water at 90%. If you increase the 4 lbs. by 20%, you will know you need approximately 4.8 lbs. of starting product. Therefore, a person who weighs 130 obs. needs to eat up to 5 lbs. of fruit. If you feel that this amount is too much for you just eat as much as you can without pushing yourself too much. It is recommended to eat at least 30 g. (1oz.) of parsley. The rest of the greens, dill, green onion, lettuce, etc. you can eat as much as you want.
5. During the day you can either stay with one type of fruit or combine a few different types. Depending on the season, you can change the types and combination of fruits.
6. With decreased acidity of stomach juices and with candida, use sour types of fruit. With increased acidity of stomach juices, it is better to use sweet or sour-sweet types.

Cleansing from Heavy Metals

The lymph cleansing techniques with fresh fruit not only cleanses the lymph, but it has other great benefits as well.

If chewed properly, juicy fruits quickly release a large amount of juices, which can be absorbed rapidly. The remaining fiber, as it passes through digestive tract, also has a number of positive effects.

- Finely broken down fiber *prevents the absorption of harmful substances.*
- Pectins of fruits and vegetables *have an ability to collect salts of heavy metals,* **lead, cobalt, mercury, chromium, nickel, copper** *and others, and remove those from the body.*
- Hard strands of fiber *"brush off" dirt, mucus and stones from walls of the intestine.*
- All of the fruits and vegetables used for this cleansing, have slight laxative properties, *which helps in cleansing the digestive system: stomach, small intestine, and large intestine.*

At only age 59 was very sick.

High Blood Pressure, high sugar, swollen leg and weight of **285 lb.**
My Aunt and cuisine told me about this Russian doctor and his staff and all the wonders they experienced in the Koyfman Whole Body Cleansing.
I came in for my first visit on May 26, 2004. After only sixteen treatments I weighed **222 lb.** I stopped taking sugar pills. My blood pressure is much lower and my blood pressure medication was reduced two times. My joints are not swollen I don't get water retention any more and don't feel bloated. Feels like all of my body systems are functioning much better. This is so much more than I ever expected. I am amazed. I am rejuvenated. **I am alive again!**
I want to thank my aunt, cuisine, the doctor and God for sending me this way.   **- - - Roy B.   August 11, 2004**

The Wonder Cleanse!

After having my Small Intestine Cleansing procedure done I felt tremendous results. I came in with a cold and left without it. Later I noticed that my chronic headache was gone. My digestion has improved.

I have suffered from arthritis for many years and now my joints do not hurt, I feel more flexible and I am able to exercise again. Because my health is so much better, my mood is better as well. Because of all my chronic pains I felt miserable all the time and now that it is gone, I can actually enjoy life. My diet has changed as well. I never thought that eating healthy and even juice fasting can be so easy, interesting and enjoyable. Thank you Koyfman Center for giving me my life back.

- - - Margaret S.   Age 55

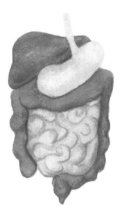

Sexual Organs

Cleansing the Prostate, Uterus, Ovaries, and Bladder

The sexual organs are the prostate (in men), the uterus and ovaries (in women), and the bladder (everyone). The pelvic area where our sexual organs are located is also home to some of the most important energetic centers (chakras).

Difficulties sometimes occur in the pelvic area when circulation is hindered and blockages occur due to chemical and biologic toxicity, sedentary lifestyles, and emotional stress. Circulation is also disrupted by raw physical pressure from nearby organs that have become enlarged due to toxins and gasses swelling them beyond their normal size. This is particularly true of the large intestine, and to a lesser (but

59

significant) degree from other organs. When swollen by accumulated solid and gaseous wastes, the walls of the large intestine are stretched thin, and toxins and bacteria more easily leak into other, nearby organs. This is a source of chemical toxicity.

Disruption of circulation and the presence of toxicity in the pelvic area can cause illnesses such as: fibroids, impotency, prostate cancer, menstrual irregularities, inability to have children, bladder inflammation and etc. That's why to prevent diseases of the organs in this area it is important to prevent the build-up of toxicity and protect against blood circulation being disrupted.

Methods of Cleansing the Sexual Organs

• Removing toxicity in the body, and the pressure on organs in the pelvic area that comes with the toxicity.
• Cleansing the blood.
• Removing residual stress and emotional tensions.
• Reestablishing normal circulation of both blood and energy in the organs and glands located in the pelvic area.

Now let's figure out which of the things listed above you can do by yourself, and where you would need the help of a professional.

To Remove Toxicity and Pressure

1. Cleanse the large intestine (under a practitioner's care).
2. Cleanse the small intestine (under a practitioner's care).

3. Switch to a cleansing diet such as described in the book *Deep Internal Body Cleansing,* and do not overload the stomach with too much food.

To Cleanse the Blood

1. Cleanse the liver 4-5 times (under a practitioner's care).
2. Cleanse the lymph (under a practitioner's care).
3. Adhere to the principles of correct diet described in *Unique Method of Colon Rejuvenation.*
4. Drink fresh vegetable juices (include greens, beet root, and 1-2 cloves of garlic).

To Remove Sources of Emotional Stress in These Organs

1. Cleanse the stomach, liver, small intestine (under a practitioner's care).
2. Get an internal organ massage (under a practitioner's care).
3. Practice meditation and conscious relaxation of internal organs. (This requires that you first study that with a professional, and then will be able to meditate by yourself.)

To Re-Establish Normal Circulation of Both Blood and Energy

1. Learn and continue special exercises (described below).
2. Do daily special self-massage (described below).

Exercises for Cleansing the Sexual Organs

The therapeutic benefit of all these exercises is an increase in blood flow in the pelvic area which in turn increases oxygenation to all of the organs, tissues, etc., in the immediate area. By increasing circulation not only of the blood, but of lymph fluids as well, you can also increase the removal of waste products from the tissues and organs, which may prevent and even help to heal some disorders in those organs.

Squeezing the Buttocks

This odd-sounding exercise can be performed while lying on your back, sitting or standing. *Without using your hands,* squeeze both sides of your buttocks toward the center using only the muscles in your rear end. Hold this tension for a few seconds and then release. At first your breathing can be regular, however, when you become more familiar with this simple exercise you should squeeze your buttocks during exhalation. In this case hold the tension while holding your breath, and release as you inhale. Repeat the exercise 10 - 30 times. The **therapeutic effects** of this exercise include helping with **hemorrhoids and diseases of the colon.**

Tightening the Sexual Nerve

Sit in a straight-backed chair, or in any yoga pose, with your legs crossed. While slowly inhaling, squeeze the sexual nerve (the area between the reproductive organs and anus), and pull it upward so that in men testis rise and in women ovaries rise up. After holding the squeeze for a second, relax and exhale slowly. Repeat the exercise 10-20 times. The **therapeutic**

effect of this exercise is to **improve the growth and function of the reproductive organs.**

Attention Gentlemen: The lack of proper blood circulation in the pelvic area can lead to disruptions in functioning of the testis and the prostate glands. Problems resulting from poor circulation include:

• Loss of clear thinking.
• Early gray hair.
• Impotence.

For men, the therapeutic benefits of increasing blood circulation in the pelvic area include clearer thinking, longer lasting youthful hair color, and improved sexual energy and enjoyment.

Attention Ladies: The lack of proper blood circulation in the pelvic area can lead to disruptions in functioning of the uterus and the ovaries. Problems resulting from poor circulation include:

• Problems with the nervous system.
• Menstrual irregularities.
• Low blood pressure.
• Mispositioning of the uterus.
• Infertility.

For women, the therapeutic benefits of increasing blood circulation in the pelvic area include a balanced nervous system, menstrual ease, regulated blood pressure, proper uterus position, and normalized fertility.

Tightening the Sexual and Anal Nerves Simultaneously

Sit in a straight-backed chair, or in any yoga pose, with your legs crossed. Inhale moderately and pull your stomach in. Tighten the sexual and anal nerve (the anus) at the same time while holding your breath for 3-5 seconds. Relax and exhale at the same time. Repeat the exercise 15-20 times. The **therapeutic effects** include **strengthening the testes and the prostate.** If you do this exercise while having a bowel movement, you can stimulate elimination and better cleansing of the colon.

Other Exercises for Improving Circulation in the Area

There are several exercises discussed in my book *Unique Method of Colon Rejuvenation.* These are referenced here: exercises 4, 6, and 7. All three of these exercises massage all the internal organs in the whole area. They improve circulation, provide cleansing and nourishment, and strengthen these organs.

Yoga has a variety of other beneficial exercises for the organs in this area. Also, notice that even such a simple exercise as walking around on all fours, i.e. simulating animals, is also very good for organs in the pelvic area.

Giving a Helping Hand to Hemorrhoids

Admittedly, this is not a topic to be lightly discussed at your next soiree, but if you are having misery sitting down or passing stools, the information here can be valuable.

Hemorrhoids are caused when hard, dry stools pass through the rectum. As these pass, the extra friction of these dry wastes tugs on the tender inner lining at the end of the colon, and pulls it down and out. It is no surprise therefore that this tissue is very sensitive.

What is often not known is that hemorrhoids have varicose veins due to the trauma of being pulled out of place. This means that blood vessels become clogged with toxins and other wastes. One avenue of relief comes from self-massaging these tender tissues to increase circulation and cause wastes trapped in these blood vessels to move on.

Before we go any further, it should be mentioned that this specific self-massage recommends the use of medical grade rubber gloves. They are sanitized to prevent contamination, and they are lightweight enough to allow you to feel what you are doing. Protecting yourself from the germs always found under fingernails is important, as is isolating your hands from any minute amounts of waste that may still be in this area. When the gloves are lightly coated with a massage oil or olive oil all friction is removed, and one can still feel what is being done.

To perform this massage, put on one pair of rubber gloves, and then lubricate the finger tips of the gloves as described above. Reach back to the area with the hemorrhoids with only one hand and begin to massage around the affected area. Begin very gently, and literally feel your way through the process. (Because the hemorrhoids are on the outside of the rectum, there is no need to insert your fingers inside the rectum.)

The basic idea is to stroke the hemorrhoids along the length of the veins in the hemorrhoids so that wastes are pushed out and circulation is increased. Once the toxins are back in circulation, the blood stream will take them to the liver and kidneys for processing and removal. The increase in circulation caused by the massage will speed healing.

You will know when you are massaging this area correctly. It is really a matter of intuition, especially since this area is not one easily observed. Once you have completed the massage on the first side, switch hands and do the other side if needed. Even if not needed, a massage in this second area is beneficial.

When finished, pull the gloves off inside out. This traps any wastes on the gloves inside when you throw the gloves away. Gloves should only be used one time. Never re-use gloves employed in this fashion. Also, watch for any allergic reaction to the material from which the gloves are made. It is rare, but it does happen, that a rash will develop on the skin of the hands from wearing rubber or latex gloves. If one gets a rash on the hands, you can be sure that this material is not beneficial for other parts of the body.

Another way to perform this massage is in the shower. In this case one can use soap as a lubricant and accomplish a more thorough cleansing at the same time. Some people choose not to use rubber gloves in this situation because the soap is protecting the anal area and their hands from significant contamination. When finished, the rectal area should be well-flushed with water from the shower, and the hands should be thoroughly cleaned, especially under the fingernails.

If you do this simple technique properly and regularly each time you take a shower, you may prevent or even heal hemorrhoids for yourself.

Strengthening the Anal Muscles and Whole Body Rejuvenation

In our practice, during the colon cleansing procedure, we often meet with a phenomena in which a client's anal muscle is so weak that it is unable to hold tightly the inserted speculum. As a result, during the procedure, water flows around the speculum onto the table. Weakened anal muscles can create other unpleasant accidents for an individual. With a sneeze, cough, or passing of gas, the large intestine may unexpectedly release fecal matter.

Why Does It Happen?

Accumulation of toxins and excess gas in the large intestine create enormous pressure on the rectum and anus. Straining in the restroom during elimination adds pressure on the vessels and anal muscles. As a result, vessels in that area expand and push out through the muscle tissue (called hemorrhoids), and also the muscle itself becomes weakened.

Eastern medicine believes that by the strength or weakness of the anal muscle, you can diagnose the biological age of a person. The weaker anal muscle is, the older the person is biologically. This means that 35-year-old person with a weak anal muscle could have a biological age of 65-70, and vice versa. If an elderly individual has strong anal muscles, his or her biological age may be 20-30. Anal muscles can be strengthened by cleansing, exercise, and self-massage, as described earlier. By doing this exercise regularly, it will not only free you of discomfort associated with a weak anus, but also improve your sexual performance, rejuvenate your whole body and reverse your age.

Cleansing the Prostate Gland with Massage

There are two basic kinds of massage for the prostate. The first is "through the rectum," and should only be performed by a professional trained in this technique. This particular massage directly touches the prostate, and should not be performed by someone who has no training.

The second technique is the self-massage, and avoids the rectum completely. It is less direct, but has great benefit nonetheless. Using one hand at a time, or both hands simultaneously, gently grab the tissue of the uppermost inner thigh immediately adjacent to the sex organs. Begin massaging this area very gently at first, and increase the strength of the massage as it feels correct. Be careful not to apply too much pressure since any massage can be overdone.

As you massage this area you should move further inward toward the sex organs and massage all around them. (For this massage, do not massage the sex organs themselves.) Gently reach into the tissues in this area with your fingertips while consciously thinking how your technique is increasing circulation. Remember not to do this too hard for this is a sensitive area. The amount of time necessary should be at least one minute. Again, you should feel your way through this self-massage.

This massage can be done in the shower or while soaking in a hot tub. It is particularly satisfying when kneeling in a warm or hot tub of water. (Pick your perfect temperature.) The hot water increases circulation even further.

Therapeutic Benefits of this Massage

- Helps to cleanse the prostate.
- Prevents prostate disorders.
- Increases sexual energy.
- When used together with other cleansing procedures, diet, and exercises, this massage may help to heal prostate disorders.

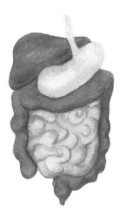

Joints and Spine

When a child is born its joints are very flexible, but with age this flexibility decreases. This happens because the modern, busy person does not use the full range of movement potential in his joints and spine. In some joints a person uses only 30-40 percent of the full range of motion. As a result, the circulation in the unused portion decreases, allowing the accumulation of toxins in the form of uric acid crystals which stick to the bones in the joints.

Where many such crystals have accumulated, the joints can retain water, and the soft tissue around such joints becomes filled with excessive amounts of fluid. The tissue around these joints becomes swollen, and the crystals on the bones rip and tear these tissues with their sharp edges. This causes extreme pain. Humidity and rain prevent the evaporation of excess water through the skin and kidneys. During this kind of weather, the tissues swell up even more and cause what's known as "weather pains."

Intense, prolonged, or frequent stress on the joints also has negative effects and can be the cause of arthritis. During prolonged stress on the joint, there is the possibility of disruption in lubrication with sinovial fluid. If there is not enough of sinovial fluid, the bones in the joint start rubbing against each other and wear down. Runners, pianists, masseurs, and people in other professions which require stress on joints can develop arthritis in middle and older age.

Another reason for problems in the joints is an excessive consumption of animal protein and fat. This diet in conjunction with a sedentary lifestyle promotes the formation of uric acid crystals. People who are vata type are more susceptible to problems with joints than people who are pita or kafa types.

Methods of Maintaining Joints in Conditions of Full Movement and Absence of Pain

Exercises

The best exercises are those from yoga and walking. Long walks, up to one hour in length, provide a good method of toning all joints. In addition, yoga exercises are very effective in keeping joints healthy. It is important to find a knowledgeable and experienced yoga teacher so that the exercises prove beneficial rather than harmful. However, do not be afraid of yoga exercises; there are so many of them that you can always chose the ones that you can do safely. When performing any exercises try to stay in the range of your abilities, not going to extremes. There should be no pain or excessive pressure. Flexibility and strength come slowly, with regular training. Yoga exercises allow you to use your joints in the most appropriate range of motions.

Mind Exercises

For people who have serious problems with their joints, who find it difficult to move or who cannot move at all, it is best to start with visualization, massage, baths, and training only in the range which is comfortable. Short training sessions of 5-10 minutes should be performed 2-5 times a day.

Visualization, or we can call it "mind joint exercise," is performed in the following way:

1. Sit in a comfortable chair.
2. Close your eyes.
3. Relax your muscles and slow down your breathing by concentrating and looking "within."
4. You should do this in silence.
5. Imagine yourself, or if that's too hard imagine somebody else, performing joint exercises. See the explanation on how to perform these exercises in the chapter entitled, "Instructions for Joint Cleansing," in my book, *Eight Steps to Perfect Health*
6. You should see the exercise through all of its movements.
7. Count the number of repetitions. There should be 10 or more repetitions in those joints where you have a problem.
8. In your mind's eye move from joint to joint, seeing the exercises connected with each joint.
9. Imagine all of the possible movements: turns, bends, spins, etc.
10. To understand better what you should imagine, try first to do each movement physically, but very gently, or, if

71

you cannot do them, ask your friend to do them for you.

If you can't clearly see these images, then just think about these exercises. That in itself should yield some results.

Therapeutic Benefits of Mind Exercises

When you consciously make yourself think or see these exercises in your mind, **you activate the centers in the brain which are responsible for these movements.** Those brain centers, weakened through lack of use but now activated, trigger the work of the nerves (also weakened from lack of use) through which signals are sent to muscles and joints. **Exercises in the mind also activate circulation in the joint which you picture at work.** If you were to perform these mental exercises regularly enough, you would be able to "order" their performance while you are sleeping. You could program yourself to dream about doing joint exercises or about running.

In addition to mind exercises, it is necessary, if you are able, to go on to perform the actual movements and exercises to improve circulation in your joints. If you are persistent you will definitely succeed, especially if you can go through the course of cleansing procedures.

Diet and Juice Therapy

Diet plays an important role in maintaining the health of your joints. During the summer, it is best to eat more fresh raw fruits and vegetables and their juices. During the winter, you can eliminate or reduce the amount of fruit eaten, and you can steam part of your vegetables. It is best to reduce the general amount of meat products, and the best time to eat them at all is in the winter. You can eat nuts, seeds, whole grains, and fresh greens. To find out about correct combinations of food products, best time for digestion during a day, how to keep products from becoming spoiled and infested with parasites, which juices to drink to help remove crystals from joints and spine, look in my books, *Deep Internal Body Cleansing* and *Eight Steps to Perfect Health.*

Baths and Massage

Baths with sea salt or other salts are very good for the joints. You can add 3-4 cups of salt to a bath. This concentration of salt pulls out the toxins through the skin. Hot water warms the joints and activates the blood flow. This kind of bath can be done 1-2 times a week or every day.

It's also useful to do a self-massage with a dry brush. Take some extra time massaging the joints, especially the ones which cause problems.

Try to Avoid Staying Very Long in Damaging Conditions

Some conditions are very dangerous for affected joints. These conditions create negative energy which damages the whole system and creates pain in the joints and in other parts of the body. Avoid these conditions:
• Living or staying very long in a room with mold and excessive moisture.
• Staying in a moist, cold place. (Joints like dryness and heat.)
• Standing or sitting with feet on cement.
• Staying outside in cold, wet, or windy weather.

Prostate and Joints

My wife and I started the Whole Body Cleansing with Dr. Koyfman for several different reasons.

All my life I suffered from sinus infections. Two or three years ago I started having prostate problems and urinary tract infections. My blood pressure was always elevated, 130/90. After meals I felt tired and sleepy.

After only 3 visits with Dr. Koyfman, my prostate pain is completely gone! My blood pressure is 120/80. I feel energized! No more antibiotics for urinary tract infections. My breathing is getting better and my sinuses are finally clearing up. I am only 32 years of age and felt like I was falling apart. My sex drive was down to zero and I felt like an old man. Now I feel like I am sixteen again. My business is improving because I can do so much more.

My wife has severe arthritis. She is only 29, but could barely walk and move around. After only a few visits, she feels a huge difference. She has less joint pain. Her knees, feet and hands are not swollen any more. She can move easier and has more flexibility. Her mood is of course much better and she looks forward to more results!

Thanks to the Koyfman Center we can enjoy our love life, our marriage, and our 9-year-old son who has been used to seeing his parents sick for such a long time.

- - - Carlos and Adriana G. - - -

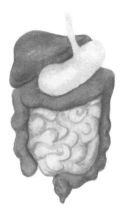

Water, Exercise, and Cleansing

The combination of water and exercise can create a powerful cleansing action, especially if you add to the water some juices or herbs which increase the cleansing action.

Water and Solutions

Before you begin your exercise routine, drink 1-2 glasses of warm water mixed with your choice of freshly squeezed lemon juice, organic apple vinegar, or a cleansing herbal tea. Lemon juice, apple vinegar, and cleansing herbs are solvents of the body's refuse. (By the way, distilled water dissolves better than any other kind.)

When we drink 1-2 large glasses of water, we temporarily increase the amount of blood and lymph circulating in the body. Additionally, blood and lymph become thinner, flow faster and more easily, and can now penetrate the smaller vessels (the capillaries) better. Thanks to thin blood and lymph penetrating the smaller vessels more deeply, the area that can be cleansed increases. The refuse on the walls of vessels and cells is routed to the excretory channels, the kidneys, skin, lungs, and the large intestine.

Exercises

After you drink the water, start your exercises. While doing the exercises, continue drinking water or cleansing tea, but now in small doses of one or two gulps each, every five minutes. If, while exercising, you feel the need to "go," then go, and when you come back, continue the exercises.

If one of the excretory channels—for example the large intestine—is blocked, the other excretory organs, lungs, kidneys, and skin, will do the bulk of the work. If this happens, it is time for you to take measures to unblock the large intestine, i.e., colon hydrotherapy.

Your wellness is an indicator of the state of your excretory channels. If, while exercising and after exercising, you feel excellent, your excretory channels are healthy. But if you feel worse, it means one or more of the following:

• That you have a high level of toxicity.
• That you exercise too vigorously.
• That one or more of your excretory organs is blocked, i.e., can't cope with all the toxins trying to pass through.

Breathing

During and after exercising, it is wise to perform breathing exercises. If you perform your exercises correctly, breathing becomes deeper on its own. After exercising, you need to do several breathing exercises, or better yet go for a walk which will also stimulate your breathing automatically.

As a result of the breathing exercises, the body receives more oxygen. Oxygen helps neutralize toxins that were released from the vessels and cells. The liver also plays a role in neutralizing the toxins; thus you should periodically massage and heat the liver during exercises.

If You Feel Worse Instead of Better

If, after the physical and breathing exercises, not all released toxins are removed from the blood and lymph, your sense of wellness can become worse: you may feel weakness, nausea, and other symptoms. To prevent this, keep your excretory channels clean. You already know how to do that. But if you still get worse, you should sit down, or better yet, lie down on your back, close your eyes, relax all the muscles in your body and stay perfectly still for 5-10 minutes. This will help calm your circulation, and detached refuse will settle and stick again. Blood and lymph will become cleaner and you will feel better. You will fell freshness, calmness, and an influx of energy.

After this complex of treatments, if you did everything right, the total amount of refuse in your body will be decreased. Part of the energy of the body's defenses will be freed from the battle against toxins, and this released energy will be used to increase your vitality. You will feel more capable, more determined and stronger. Occasionally you may feel seemingly causeless influxes of joy. Of course, however, there is a reason. The reason lies not in joyful events, but in the lack of the harmful influence of toxins on the body. **The feeling of pleasure from life is always present in a cleansed organism.**

To learn more about unique cleansing procedures done in our center, please visit our website at
www.koyfmancenter.com

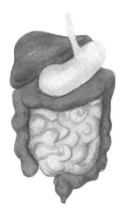

Negative Emotions

The Effects of Negative Thoughts and Emotions on the Body

Frequently repeated negative thoughts and emotions can cause tension in muscles and organs so that they tighten up like a frightened animal trying to hide from danger. After the stress has passed, these tensions do not completely disappear but leave behind a "residue"of stress. Unfortunately, these residues can build up with each significant incident.

Problems from this build-up of tension take several different forms. For example, the tension in muscles and organs uses up some of the energy of the body, weakening its immune system.

This constant but low-grade tension also contributes to blockages that hinder the circulation of nutrients, blood, lymph, oxygen, energy, etc. Blockages and reduction of internal circulation disrupt the processes of digestion and of cleansing the organs and cells. For example:

- Blockages in the digestive system slow down the movement of food through the digestive tract. Food stays in the areas of tension longer than necessary, allowing for the beginning of such processes as fermentation, putrefication, gas formation and poisoning via toxification.
- Blockages in the respiratory system disrupt the cells' saturation with oxygen and off-loading of carbon dioxide.
- Blockages and tensions in the circulatory system disrupt the work of the heart, may cause hypertension, weaken the blood vessels, disrupt the delivery of nutrients to the cells, and prevent cell cleansing.

Tension and blockages in different organs and muscles prevent them from functioning normally. Problems such as "energy leaks," deficient nutrient and oxygen delivery, excessive levels of toxins, etc. occur. In a weakened body, favorable conditions are created for the growth of various bacteria, parasites, and diseases. Blockages in the circulatory system strain the heart which causes it to become overworked and wear down faster.

Stress from negative emotions promotes an increased secretion of hormones into the blood. In natural stress situations, such as "fight or flight" physical danger, a person uses up these hormones through increased physical activity such as running, fighting, or working. These hormones are burned up by the muscles, and do not cause harm.

However, in today's social settings, negative emotions are usually not acted upon physically. Therefore, your anger stays inside of you. The large amounts of hormones secreted— instead of being burned off by muscles or used in digestion—

attack and harm various organs. Suppressed or unrealized emotions are the reason for the unbalance in different organs. Examples follow.

- Unexpressed anger completely changes the flora in the bladder, urethra, and small intestine. It causes inflammation of mucus membranes of the stomach and small intestine.
- Unexpressed fear affects many organs including the large intestine, changing its flora. As a result you feel bloated from excess of gas, which accumulates in the folds of large intestine and causes pain.
- Depression and sadness create tensions and blockages in the lungs.
- Fear attacks the kidneys and heart.
- Anxiety and nervousness affect the stomach and spleen.
- Anger disrupts functions of the liver and bladder, increases blood pressure, and can result in a heart attack.
- Impatience and hastiness create tensions and disrupt circulation in the heart.
- The small intestine is an universal organ for collecting the dregs of all the negative emotions, because in its many parts all of them can find a place, fear in the lower right part, anger in the upper right, worry in the upper middle, caretaking in the upper left, and sadness in the lower left.

Negative emotions can transform from one kind into another kind. Sadness can change into depression, worry into impatience, impatience into anger, unexpressed anger into hurt. As a result, large amounts of secreted and unused hormones drawn out by negative emotions poison the body. On the other hand, these hormones are fuel for the production of large amounts of energy, which we suppress to our own harm. Is it possible to learn to change our actions in such a way that the secreted hormones of negative emotions would work for our benefit and not to harm us?

Techniques for Slowing Negative Emotions and Transforming Their Energy Toward Useful Action

Let's first examine situations of extreme emotion. These situations result in the formation of strong negative stress. In these circumstances, if you know and remember what to do, you can create a reliable barrier and then gradually, completely eliminate all of the effects of this harmful situation.

So, let's examine every step. During a situation of extreme negative emotion there are a lot of hormones secreted into blood. Heartbeat increases, breathing becomes harder, muscles become tense, and vessels constrict.

At this point you need to learn to observe yourself emotionally and physically in order to quickly and accurately determine that you are experiencing extreme stress. As soon as you determine that; take a slow deep breath in, a normal breath out, and then hold your breath for as long as you can. In 10-15 seconds, your **body** will realize that it has another problem—namely a of lack of oxygen—and that the stress level is lower. Your **body** focuses on the more serious problem. Your **mind** might still be focused on the problem of stress, but your subconscious has already registered the breathing problem as a life-threatening condition and has started to act accordingly.

At first the most important body action is to make available to the brain the rest of the oxygen present in the body. To achieve that, the body dilates blood vessels, facilitating the transport to the brain of the unused oxygen in the lungs and in the blood. The heart slows down and starts to work more efficiently. Muscle tension decreases. With this technique, the level of stress is reduced. Now you can think and act more logically.

When you feel that you are approaching your breath holding limit start slowly inhaling through the nose. For awhile try not to breathe very deeply, which will allow vessels to stay dilated.

Now all you have to do is to choose a type of activity which will be good for you to use up secreted hormones. Quickly decide what kind of active work you need (not sitting or sedentary). Clean your house or office, gather leaves in the yard, rearrange your furniture, or whatever works for you. The choices of useful activity to use up the energy of secreted hormones depends on where you are, what needs to be done, and what you might prefer to do at the moment, etc. If you have a chance to go for a long walk or jogging, it will be very beneficial.

If you are in a place where you can't perform any kind of physical activity, repeat the breath holding after exhalation, giving yourself a three-minute break between repetitions. Also, you can flex different muscles of your body (legs, buttocks, shoulders, arms, jaws, etc.) and keep them flexed for 5-10 seconds; then give yourself a break and repeat the flexing until you feel a little tired.

In fact, all kinds of activities for using up the energy of secreted hormones should be performed until you feel a light to moderate level of tiredness. Tiredness and absence of repeating thoughts tells you that you have used up all of the excess hormones.

Other Methods of Removing the Effects of Stress from Your Body

During stress, the muscles which are most tense are those of the shoulders, back of the neck, face, and forehead. Even without having special knowledge, you can "read" a person's face to figure out if he is sad, nervous or angry. Dropped shoulders and neck say that a person is fearful. Tension in the shoulders gets passed on to the hands, and if you observe hands you can also tell if the person is nervous or calm. Voice, manner of speaking, and breathing also gives us information about another person's emotions.

Depending on where physical tensions are located, you can choose a method of removing them. For example:

- Tension in the shoulders can be relieved by exercises which involve the shoulder, and by massaging the shoulders.
- Tension in the face is relieved with exercises for face muscles, massage, and methods of thought control.
- Tension and nervousness in the voice can be removed through breathing exercises, relaxation and thought control.

Chi Machine Method

You can use a chi machine to release stress tensions and the blockages that form in the regions of these tensions.

Technique of Chi Machine Usage

Use this method in the morning on an empty stomach or in the evening before supper. Ten minutes before you start, drink a large glass of water with lemon juice. Drinking a cup of water before the session increases the blood volume in the blood system. This brings more blood to tension areas and helps to break up the blockages. Don't forget to empty your bladder and, if possible, your colon.

1. You may turn on quiet, calming music if you wish.
2. Set the chi machine timer for 10-15 minutes.
3. Lie on your back on a carpet.
4. Place your ankles on the chi machine.
5. Place your arms parallel to your body, and close your eyes.

Use of the chi machine produces rhythmic vibrational movements of the body which shake and relax all the muscles and organs of your body. These movements are similar to the movements of a fish, and happen without any effort *whatsoever* from you. They are repeated thousands of times during a single session, relaxing you more and more deeply.

Because the entire body is involved in these movements, all your muscles and organs gain relaxation in this method. The relaxing effect can be further increased if you consciously concentrate your attention on specific organs and muscles and give them *orders* to relax and calm down.

Pay special attention to relaxing your eyes, muscles of your forehead, cheeks, neck, and thyroid gland. Then you need to examine and feel out the muscles of your legs, arms, and trunk, and then your internal organs, stomach, pancreas, small intestine, kidneys, lungs, backbone, etc. Examine all organs and muscles in your body, and pay special attention to those that bother you. Concentrating your attention on your muscles and organs allows them to relax even more completely.

Against the background of this relaxation and passivity in the body, there is also further relaxation in the widening of the large blood vessels and the opening of capillaries. In this way, the flow of blood, lymph, and energy in your organism intensifies and accelerates as tension is reduced.

Then, as the session ends, a phenomenal and important combination of events occurs. Just before the machine turns off, all your organs are relaxed and passive while inside of you, the movement of blood, lymph, and energy accelerates as relaxation increases. At the moment when the chi machine stops, another important phenomenon occurs. The body complete stops moving, as the car might feel if you pushed the brakes to the metal, but the internal movements continue. The universal law of momentum snaps into action. It tears the tensions and blockages from their accustomed places. Intense circulation of energy and body fluids begins in those areas, and you may experience certain intense feelings at this moment.

Move your attention to the spot where you feel the greatest vibration of energy, and keep it there until the feeling weakens. The region where you feel the strongest vibrations is the region where a breakthrough of energy has occurred, and usually in that area is your main problem at this time. Tension here has been released as the momentum knocked the blockages from their places. Energy channels opened and blood, lymph, and energy started flowing through a region that was previously closed to them and started to clean toxins from cells and to supply them with nutrients. **Notice: the process of breaking up blockages and tensions in organs happens more effectively after deep internal body cleansing.**

Try to imagine at this time how tensions loosen and blockages leave your body. This will aid the processes of cleansing your body of negative emotions.

Of course, not all blockages and tensions will disappear after only one session. Over the course of your life, hundreds or even thousands of these blockages collect in your organism. Regular, daily sessions with the chi machine are necessary. It might be that several months or a year would be necessary to remove all tensions and blockages, but with every session, you will feel better and better.

The Method of Positive Suggestion and the Internal Smile

Imagine your body as a vessel. The vessels contents always have an influence on the vessel. If you fill it with pure water, the vessel will not be harmed in any way, but instead, it will be purified. If you fill the vessel with sulphuric acid, it will be burned. If you fill your body vessel with toxins, negative thoughts and emotions, this volatile concoction will sear and upset it no matter how much you try to strengthen the body vessel with exercises.

Let's take a look at what thoughts and emotions fill a modern person. Constant hurry, fear of being late, work problems, family problems, worrying about children, low esteem for yourself and others, offenses, fear of the future, frustrations, jealousy, irritation, etc. The caustic mixture of negative thoughts and emotions destroys the body like rust. A huge number of nerves passes through the body, connecting the brain with every organ and every cell. Every thought generated in the brain immediately passes through the nerves to every cell. Negative information suppresses and upsets the functioning of cells.

Words also play a great role in the influence the brain exerts on the organs. There are people who constantly talk about their maladies. Whoever the meet, thcy explain all the details about their diseases, surgeries, drugs. They indulge in telling how bad they slept, where they had pain, that nothing helps, etc. Instead of doing something worthwhile to help the body, they find pleasure in trying to elicit pity for themselves with their tales. If you tell your friends—and you think about yourself in your mind that you are ill, weak, and old—a hundred times per day, you make your organs sit through it a hundred times per day. The information they receive is negative self-suggestion. With such destructive self-programming, you upset your body so much that no treatment will ever help you, unless you quit filling your body with toxic thoughts, emotions, and words.

In Daoism, negative emotions are considered low-quality energy. This energy is destructive and leads to disease.

High-quality energy is creative and can cure diseases. It can be produced by an internal smile to all parts of your body, to all organs, glands, and muscles. By smiling to your organs, you force them to become relaxed, soft, and calm. By smiling to your vessels, you cause them to relax and expand.

The practice of the internal smile should begin with the eyes. The eyes are the connection to the vegetative, or autonomic, nervous system, which controls the functioning of glands and other organs. The eyes are the first to receive frightening emotional signals and influence the glands through the nerves, forcing them to make stress-producing hormones. Then when the critical situation passes, the eyes send to the organs the signals for relaxation. By relaxing your eyes, you can relax your whole body.

Technique of the Internal Smile

When you are only beginning the practice, find a quiet spot where nobody will bother you. After you have gained experience, you will be able to practice this technique anywhere.

It is best to do this on an empty stomach or at least two hours after a meal.

1.   Sit comfortably at the edge of a chair. Put your hands on you knees. Close your eyes. Breathe normally.

2.   Relax your forehead. Feel the smiling energy in your eyes.

3.   Move the smiling energy to your face and cheeks. Feel how it spreads and warm your cheeks.

4.   Move the smiling energy to the tip of your tongue, and then feel how it fills the whole tongue. Touch your top mandible with your tongue and leave your tongue in that position for the rest of the session.

5.   Move the smiling energy to your neck. The neck often harbors many tensions. These stresses lessen the circulation in the brain and the thyroid gland. Smile to the front and rear surfaces of your neck and feel how it is cleansed and relaxed.

6.   Smile to your thyroid gland, which protects you. Feel how it opens like a flower. Tell yourself: *My thyroid is healthy. It perfectly performs all of its functions and is a formidable defense against all my enemies.*

7.   Return your attention to your eyes and increase their smiling energy.

8.   Move the smiling energy to your heart. The heart is an organ that works nonstop throughout your entire life. Feel the smiling energy in the heart, how your heart is relaxed and calm. Thank your heart for its labor. Say in your mind: *My heart works rhythmically, calmly and*

correctly. My heart is absolutely healthy. All my vessels are healthy and clean. I am perfectly calm.

9.   Return your attention to your eyes, and again increase their smiling energy.

10.   Move the smile to your lungs. The lungs supply the body with oxygen and remove carbon dioxide. Feel how smiling energy relaxes your lungs. Imagine how the lungs reply to the smile of your eyes with their own smile. Say in your mind: *My breathing is light and calm. I am totally calm and relaxed.*

11.   Once again, return your attention to your eyes and feel how the smiling energy in them surges. This happens because now a large number of your organs are smiling, increasing the combined smile of your body, which is reflected in your eyes.

12.   Now, using the same principle, move the internal smile to all other organs, the stomach, the backbone, etc. Feel their relaxation, softness, and warmth. Tell each organ that it is healthy and that it perfectly performs its functions.

By using the internal smile, you fill the vessel of your body with joy and positive suggestions. These contents strengthen the organism and program it for health and healing.

Practice the technique of the internal smile every morning after you wake up. It will give you energy for the rest of the day.

If you have little time, perform the technique faster. Pass over organs rapidly and only make slightly longer stops on the organs that bother you.

Practice the internal smile and positive suggestion when under stress. Smile to all body parts and organs in which you feel tension. Soon you will feel relaxation and softness in them, and positive suggestion will convert harmful negative energy into constructive positive energy.

If you feel pain or weakness in some organ or body part, smile longer to it. Give it a bigger dose of positive emotions. Do this until you feel better.

Conclusion: To be healthy, always monitor that with which you are filling the vessel of your body. That is, control your thoughts and emotions. (See Book 1 for the techniques of thought control.) Be sure to find time during each day to fill your body and all its organs with smiles and positive energy. Imagine and tell yourself: *I am healthy. I am calm. I am young. I am full of energy. I am love. I am forgiveness. I am goodness. I am power. I am absolutely healthy!*

The Toxic Dimension of Negative Emotions

Increased toxicity in the body leads to increased sensitivity of the nervous system to the effects of negative emotions. When your organs are not cleansed you are out of chemical balance, constantly feeling nervous and can be easily set off. Cleansing of the internal organs relieves nervousness, relaxes the nervous system, removes blockages from the organs, and removes the tensions of past stresses from the muscles.

In addition to these cleansing procedures for removing old stress tensions and blockages, and preventing new blockages, there are other methods. Let's list some of them.

List of Methods for Cleansing from Negative Emotions

Cleansing Method

- Stomach Cleansing.
- Liver Cleansing.
- Small Intestine Cleansing.
- Fasting.

Physical Method

- Breathing Exercises.
- Holding the Breath after Exhale.
- Walking with Deep Breathing.
- Any Physical Exercises and Any Physical Activity.
- Self-massage, especially face, neck, and abdominal organs.
- Chi Machine.

Heat and Water Method

- Sauna.
- Warm Bath.
- Hot and Cold Shower (changing several times).
- Swimming.
- Cold Splash (bucket of cold water).

Psychological Method

- Forgiveness.
- Relaxation.
- Meditation.
- Praying.
- Internal Smile.

The best way to get rid of negative emotions is to use combinations of these methods. Choose one or two items from each section.

Concluding Recommendation

Here is one more recommendation on how to eliminate, or at least decrease, the amount of negative emotions in your body. To give you this recommendation, I will restate some well-known truths. Repetition of these truths cannot hurt but will remind you of things you already know and might not notice in the fast pace of everyday life.

Unkind actions toward people around you create negative emotions inside you and inside of them. Such actions include carelessness, excessive pride, selfishness, jealousy, anger, arrogance, etc.

Kind actions are the sources of positive emotions for both you and others. They include thoughtfulness, good attitude, love, understanding, compassion, forgiveness, etc.

More good deeds and less bad deeds equals more positive effects and less negative effects on your body and health.

How negative emotions affect the brain and how to cleanse your brain from negative emotions are described other books of *Healing through Cleansing*. See Book 2 for a chapter on brain cleansing, and Book 1 for a chapter entitled, "The Role of the Mind."

Important Notice: Cleansing the body from negative emotions is one of the most important cleansings. In many cases without this cleansing other cleansing procedures give only temporary results.

Dr. Koyfman and my adoptive Ukrainian family

were great and a pleasure to see everyday. I arrived from Florida on April 1st, 2005 as a **250 pound** guy, who had eaten too much fast food in my life and left the clinic **20 days later** on April 21st, 2005 as a healthy **225 lb.** guy who had more energy, felt better, and with a renewed sense of life and how to live healthy. I intend to lose many more pounds, but I am confident that Dr. Koyfman has erased 22 years of poor eating and rejuvenated me internally for my next step towards a healthy lifestyle. Dr. Koyfman, his wife and son were fantastic, and Helen and Olga were a huge help through my treatment.
Eternally Greatful,   Brian L., 22

"I Highly Recommend"

I have enjoyed the experience of colonic health and feel much healthier after each procedure. The massages and saunas are also a great way to relieve stress and toxins. I highly recommend anyone at any age giving it a try.
- Briggs Allen, 35 years old

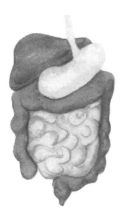

Parasites

Most Americans prefer to close their eyes to the possibility that they might somehow have parasites. Instead we prefer to believe that our technology and science, combined with our civilized personal hygiene, protect us from this seemingly foreign menace. We tend to think that parasitic infections are just a phenomenon of third world countries that have poor sanitation, etc.

However, some American doctors estimate that 85 percent of adults in North America are infected with parasites. Dr. Peter Wina, Chief of Patho-Biology at the *Walter Reed Army Institute of Research*, said in 1991, "We have a tremendous parasite problem right here in the U.S. It is just not being addressed."

While it is true that parasitic infections are a very visible health problem in some third world countries, and their governments expend great effort to educate the population about the problem, parasites are still at the root of a wide range of health concerns here in America. In fact, Dr. Frank Nova, Chief of the *Laboratory for Parasitic Diseases* at the National Institute of Health said, "In terms of numbers there are more parasitic infections acquired in this country than in Africa."

Admittedly, it is hard for us to swallow this dramatic statement, however the consensus is growing among health care professionals here that parasites are linked to numerous diseases and illnesses ranging from the insignificant all the way to cancer. So hiding one's head in the sand will not make the problem go away. It will only give the parasites more time to reproduce and cause harm to your body.

How Americans Get Parasites

It is not too hard to understand how Americans get parasites once you consider where these invaders originate. Parasites, just like toxicity, are everywhere around us. Some are light enough to ride on the wind and so enter with the air we breathe. Others float or swim in bodies of fresh water such as lakes, rivers and streams. Some species thrive on plants such as grasses, while others live on or in animals including pets. Perhaps worst of all, some parasites can be found on or in the food we eat, as described below.

The Food Vector

Americans enjoy a wide range of foods that are shipped in from nations all over the globe. These fruits, vegetables and meats are not grown, harvested, packaged or shipped under the same health regulations enforced in this country. Because of this, parasites and/or their eggs, are too often **not** washed off of foreign produce. They are able to hide under the leaves of vegetables, in the irregular surfaces of fruits, or inside meats and fish. When we bring these foods home, do we wash them with the idea of removing parasites and their eggs?

If you have ever eaten in a restaurant chances are very high that you are playing host to one or more parasites. This is because not all restaurants practice the hygiene that we hope they would. Fatigued food preparers in public eating establishments do get sloppy, or just plain in a hurry because a co-worker did not show up for work. They sometimes cut corners to keep waiting patrons from becoming disgruntled. In situations like this, food is sometimes not washed thoroughly or not cooked properly. The parasites then survive long enough to reach your intestinal tract, which is all they need.

Parasites and their eggs can survive in high and low temperatures, and then start to proliferate under favorable conditions. Many parasites have developed resistance even to antibiotics. If fish and meat are undercooked, parasites in them do not die. When they get into a person's body, they find a favorable environment to grow and reproduce.

The Air Vector

Most parasites are microscopic in size and are therefore so lightweight that the wind can easily pick them up. Once airborne, it is really just a matter of random chance if they land in or on a suitable host, animal or human.

The Water Vector

Parasites in water can enter our bodies either through the skin or through drinking. Drinking unclean water is the surest means of getting parasites since they are delivered directly to the intestine where they want to be. Conversely, cuts in or scrapes on the skin can provide water borne parasites with a means of getting into the bloodstream where they can be transported to any point in the body.

The Soil Vector

One of the things that makes soil alive is the innumerable good and beneficial organisms that live there and make the soil fertile. But just as good organisms live there so do bad organisms. By "bad" I mean single cell and multiple cell life forms that are not content to stay in the soil. Instead, they are just waiting for some four-footed animal that they can invade and call home.

Failing that preferred situation, parasites in the soil get into the bodies of birds and insects, especially mosquitoes, flies, and cockroaches. Once they enter these animals' bodies, the parasites can be transported into your house.

Of course, let's not forget that most famous and unhappy activity of some children, and that is to eat dirt. It goes without saying that dirt has the potential to have every nasty thing in it. And when children eat it they open wide the door to any and every form of contamination possible, from chemical to biological.

The Animal and Pet Vector

Dogs, cats, birds and other animals that live with people in their homes, and come into physical contact with their owners, are a source of parasitic infection. No matter how hard we try to keep our four-legged and winged friends clean, they cannot be completely protected from parasites.

Pets that live outside of our homes have innumerable ways to become infected with naturally occurring parasites, including eating plants that have parasites, eating other animals that carry parasites, drinking water from contaminated water, and being bitten by insects/arachnids that carry parasites. And, of course, pets can get parasites from other pets or animals.

Cats and dogs frequently shake themselves. This natural activity on their part to rid themselves of things in their fur is fine if done outside. However, when done inside your living and working spaces their fur, saliva, parasites and parasite eggs are thrown into the air you breathe, and onto surfaces which you will later contact, including your dinner plate.

We all love to pet our pets. Unfortunately, parasites can get onto our hands, and from there into our bodies when our unwashed hands touch our eyes, mouths, food, etc. Once on our hands, we can transmit microscopic parasites to our family, friends and co-workers. Children and the elderly are the most vulnerable.

Of course petting is not the only way in which we come into contact with our pets. Close physical contact with animals, letting them sleep in your bed, permitting them to sit in your lap, letting them lick you, allowing them into your kitchen, kissing your pets, and many other such activities open the door for parasites to enter your own body. When you think of how physically close we often get to our pets it is no surprise that we pick up parasites from them.

Some people are in the habit of kissing animals, an activity that you can even see on television. Not too long ago I was watching a show on *Animal Planet* in which a young woman was eating corn-on-the-cob with her cat. It looked really funny. The cat was pulling it her way and the woman was pulling in the opposite direction. The show host made a humorous comment: "Foolish animal doesn't know that it can contract human parasites!"

On another occasion I observed on *Animal Planet* a teenaged girl letting a dog lick the inside of her mouth repeatedly. As gross as this is to most of us, we should not deny that some others will allow this. We must also realize that we should be especially concerned for children who do not know any better, and may explore their furry friends more intimately than is prudent.

An extremely important danger of parasite infestation comes from rats, mice, cockroaches, flies and other pests that keep unwelcome company with humans and carry parasites. Rat and mice feces are particularly dangerous. The *Hanta Virus* has been found to enter the human body when dry, infected rat feces were swept up, and the dust from the sweeping was breathed into the lungs. This has been fatal.

The Personal Contact Vector

It should come as no surprise that parasites can be passed from one human to another. Any transmittal of body fluids can potentially accomplish this unhappy occurrence. This includes kissing, and any form of sex, and even handshakes. Public restrooms, door handles, elevator buttons and paper money are touched by a myriad human hands carrying contagious illnesses and sometimes parasites.

The Travel or Foreign Country Vector

Many of us take full advantage of diverse travel options made available to us by modern technology. Because of widely available airline travel that can take us to virtually any part of the world, we can go places that 100 years or even 50 years ago were not reasonably available to the average American.

With this increased capacity to travel into the exotic corners of the world comes the equally increased capacity to be

100

exposed to parasites that otherwise we would never have met. The same routes of exposure (food, animals, etc.) are at work here. More prominently, parasites can be found in drinking water that has not been properly purified.

But do not think that you have to go to some third world country to get parasites. Parasites are in every country since they truly know no political boundaries.

Where in the Human Body Do Parasites Thrive?

Once parasites enter the human body, they generally prefer to live in those areas that are weak and sick, or that are polluted with toxins from our modern, chemical world. Recent research conducted in the United States, Germany, Russia and elsewhere shows that the majority of the most serious and so-called "incurable" diseases are either caused or aided by chemical toxins in the body. This is because parasites flourish in these toxins.

Although there are a multitude of sources for these chemical pollutants, some of the major sources for Americans today are:
• Car and truck exhaust.
• Mercury from tooth fillings.
• Aerosol sprays.
• Artificial chemicals in processed food.
• The toxins that form in the body due to a poor diet and poor digestion.
• Emotional stresses that weaken the immune system.
• Overheating and overcooling of the body.
• Lack of sleep.
• Lack of proper exercise.
• And others.

Approximately 90 per cent of parasites afflicting humans live in the gastrointestinal tract. A large number of these prefer the small intestine simply because it is rich in nutrients in a highly digestible form.

The other 10 per cent are scattered throughout the human body in places in which their species are particularly suited to live. Specifically, human parasites have been, and can be, found in such organs as: the brain, heart, kidneys, liver, lungs, muscles, joints, skin, blood vessels, and even teeth.

There is no part of the human body that is safe from infestation by one or more of the many species of parasites out there. Unclean internal ecology of the body, and the weakening of its defense system, create the most favorable conditions for widespread parasite growth.

Unfortunately, parasites that infect humans are many in both kind and number. Some are single-celled organisms such as bacteria and viruses, and some are multi-celled organisms. Most are too small to see with the naked eye, but some of the worms are large enough to be seen without a microscope. In fact one species of worm can reach 20 feet in length. Some female parasite species can lay up to two million eggs a day.

Ways Parasites Harm Humans

The ways parasites harm humans are many, including toxic effects, physical damage, allergic reactions, and nutritional deficits.

Toxic Effects

The toxic effects of parasites include excreting their waste and the products of their metabolism into your digestive tract, blood, and lymph system thereby poisoning your body with their refuse. They also create toxic gasses which further poison the body. Parasites lay their eggs in your body providing a new generation of these tiny monsters to begin the cycle of parasitic toxicity all over again.

Physical Damage

Both larval and adult parasites can cause significant physical damage to our bodies as they munch on our insides. Roundworms have circular mouths surrounded by teeth that look for all the world like knives. Because they feed on human blood, they use these "knives" to cut into intestinal walls to cause bleeding. Hookworms are well named as they have little hooks to cut, poke and rip the walls of the intestine. While some parasites play the vampire by sucking our blood, others prefer tissue and are literally eating us alive. Where the damage occurs is dependent on what species of parasite a person gets since different species tend to prefer one organ or another. What species one may get is in turn dependent on exposure.

Allergic Reactions

Allergic reactions can result when parasites, their larvae and their eggs die. Their little bodies disintegrate, and if not washed out the decomposition products create a whole new level of toxicity.

Allergic reactions can also be caused by parasite waste products, and when larva move from one organ to the other.

103

Some of the symptoms include asthmatic bloody cough, skin irritation, itching, cold sweat, and pain in the heart.

Nutritional Deficits

Nutritional deficits happen because parasites eat nutrients in our food, energy our bodies have stored, and the blood that carries nutrients to all parts of our bodies. On these resources they live, develop and reproduce.

Parasites consume a very important mineral, silicon. Deficit in this mineral disrupts the connection between the brain and other organs and cells. This disruption means that the brain cannot efficiently control the work of organs and cells, and can lead to interruptions in the system and to diseases.

Parasites also consume vitamin B 12. This results in poor circulation. Parasites are not shy about consuming vitamins, minerals, enzymes, hormones, or anything that is important to human health. They don't say "Please."

Because of these activities, it is easy to see the role parasites can and do play in weakening the immune system and opening the door for disease. Parasites have been found in diseases of the teeth, gums, and digestive tract, besides contributing to the most dangerous diseases: cancer and AIDS. **A recent study in Russia showed that cancer is not a colony of malformed cells but unicellular organisms that imitate human cells!**

Some of the many symptoms of parasitic infection include:

- Constipation.
- Excessive gas.
- Skin rashes.
- Fatigue.
- Bloating.
- Bloody stool.
- Digestive problems.
- Feeling unreasonably full in the stomach.

- Grinding teeth at night.
- Nausea.
- Incessant hunger.
- Depressive headaches.

Dr. Hulda Clark, Ph. D., N. D., states that parasites **and** toxicity are involved in all illnesses.

Unicellular Parasites

The simplest unicellular parasites such as Trichomonas, chlamydia, amoeba and others are slow and terrible destroyers. The most dangerous ones are Trichomonas. Usually a person doesn't recognize their presence, but will experience weight loss, weakness, and fatigue which traditional medicine may not be able to recognize either. Parasites of all kinds are hard to diagnose with the microscope. They look a lot like blood cells. They are hard to distinguish from lymphocytes.

There are several kinds of Trichomonas: **Intestinal Trichomonas** causes swelling, polyps and ulcers. **Oral Trichomonas** locate in the oral cavity, tonsils, gums, and airways produce plaque and periodontal disease. **In human blood**, which is supposed to be sterile, it is also possible to find Trichomonas. This parasite even penetrates to the **reproductive organs**. You can become infected through sexual acts, kissing, or bathing in public baths, pools or lakes. It travels through meat, fish, vegetables, fruits, and dairy products. It travels in food utensils, underwear and public bathrooms. Cats and dogs are an especially dangerous source of Trichomonas infection.

Trichomonas is a very versatile parasite. The latest studies show that Trichomonas could be one of the reasons for cancer, having an ability to turn into cancerous cells. In 1989, in Russia it was proven that malignant tumors are a concentrated mass of the unicellular parasite Trichomonas. There is a serious and worrisome conclusion that can be drawn, that cancer is a contagious parasitic disease resulting from infection.

There is an opinion that the entire population of Earth is infected with Trichomonas, but its development is very slow in the body of a healthy person. Then when the defense mechanisms of the body are at their low points, resulting from stress, impaction and other causes, the spread of Trichomonas becomes increasingly more rapid. Nadeshda Semenova thinks that today Trichomonas is the biological enemy of humans. It resembles human cells, and it can change its shape, feeding mechanisms and respiration.

How to Limit Parasitic Infection

The question quickly becomes how one can limit the vectors, or routes, of parasitic infection. As is obvious from the above, it is impossible to avoid all parasitic infections. But does that mean that you should stop washing your hands after going to the bathroom, after holding money, or stop washing fruits and vegetables, etc.? No!

To the contrary, you should create as many handicaps for parasites trying to enter your organism as possible. To accomplish this you should remember the ways that parasites enter your body and then take every reasonable precaution to seal off those routes. One place to learn more about this subject is in my book *Deep Internal Body Cleansing*.

Once you have blocked the various means of entry to these tiny invaders, the second step is to cleanse your body of the parasites that did make it inside. Simultaneously with this second step you will eliminate the conditions under which parasites can grow, develop and reproduce. In other words, you will make your body inhospitable to parasites.

Fortunately, the process needed to make your body unfit for parasitic infestation is the same process that removes toxins from the body to greatly improve your health. This includes:

- Cleansing the large intestine and other organs of chemical and biological toxins.
- Deleting from your diet the expensive processed foods that carry so many chemical toxins that feed parasites. Eliminate such foods as sweets, dairy products, white flour, and food that is low-quality or old.
- Avoiding emotional stresses, physical exhaustion, overheating and everything else that weakens your defenses.

One of the most important conditions for keeping parasites under control is a strong immune system. If the immune system is strong, it will attack the parasites, destroy them and remove them from the body. But can we have a strong immune system in this poisoned world with its unnatural living conditions, if we don't consciously aid it?

To aid the immune system in its war on parasites one can take the following actions:

- Take those special herbs have been found to specifically attack parasites. These herbs create an environment in the human body that either kills parasites, or weakens them so much the immune system can do the rest. You can find these herbs in health food stores.
- Include in your diet an entire class of food that suppress and kill parasites. Among them are garlic, onion, black radish, and cranberry.
- Keep all your internal organs cleansed, regularly. This means that after you killed the parasites in your body with

herbs, and then removed them by cleansing the small and large intestines, you should repeat these cleansings on a regular basis. Cleansings of the large intestine should be about once a month. Dr. Norman Walker had colon cleansing every week and he lived to be 119 years old. The small intestine, the organ where the most important digestion occurs and where the most parasites reside, should be cleansed once every three months. The liver must be cleansed every 6-12 months, depending on circumstances.

Cleansing from Parasites and Preventive Measures

The most important factor preventing parasites in humans is a biological resonance in the blood created by the brain. But in order for bio-resonance therapy to work, you have to have clean blood (cleanse the liver), clean and healthy digestive system (cleanse the small and large intestine plus the stomach) and regain normal communication between brain and body. To regain that communication it is necessary to cleanse the channels connecting the brain and the body.

- Cleanse the blood and lymphatic vessels.
- Cleanse the nervous system, the channels for the transmission of brain impulses.
- Cleanse the energetic channels.
- Activate brain centers.
- Replenish silicon in the body in order to increase the ability to transmit signals.

Cleansing the blood and lymphatic vessels is achieved through the cleansing of the whole body, healthy diet and physical exercises.

Cleansing the nervous system is achieved through meditation, breathing exercises, long walks, etc.

Cleansing the energetic channels is achieved through the above-described actions and conscious concentration and relaxation of all parts of the body. The ability to relax and feel any part of the body is a way and a signal to open energetic channels. If during concentration you can easily feel a certain part of your body it means that the channels are open and that part's connection with the brain is reestablished.

Activation of brain centers occurs in all inverted yoga positions and also on a tilted board. Another method of activation is visualizing images of nature and your own health. Therefore always imagine yourself healthy and strong, able to overcome any obstacles.

Silicon is one of the main conductive elements in all radio devices. If silicon comes into the body in an artificial state (breast implants) it can cause damage, but in the natural organic state, silicon is an important element for health. Its presence in the right amount (4.7 percent) is important in a human body for creation of a good conductivity between brain and all organs and cells. A deficit of silicon (or silica) interrupts this connection. Hair and nails do not grow very well. Signals from the brain are delivered to organs in distorted form. This is a sure way to the development of disease. The reason for low levels of silicon in the body is the presence of parasites. Therefore, in order to reach a healthy level, the main goal becomes to cleanse the body from toxicity and parasites.

Personal Hygiene

To prevent or to at least decrease your chances of parasite re-infestation it is crucial to strictly follow the rules of personal hygiene. These rules include the following:

- Keep your skin clean; i.e. take showers daily using a wash cloth and a natural soap. A water filter should be attached to the shower. Once or twice a week go to a sauna. Sauna opens all your pores and cleanses tissue fluids. Steam kills external parasites and opens up sinuses, bronchi and lungs.
- Keep your house, work place and clothes clean. Change your underwear daily. Wear the clothes that correspond to the activity you are involved in and also protect your body from dirt and injuries.
- Air your room, house and office more often. Don't close your windows to the sun. A lot of parasite eggs and larva die from the sun's rays.
- Carefully clean beneath your fingernails. Surprisingly to some people, this is one of the very nastiest parts of the human body. Innumerable germs are found there, and microscopic parasites can be found there as well.

If you experience symptoms of parasite infestation, or if you are diagnosed with them through laboratory or electronic testing, **do a parasite cleansing not only for yourself but for your entire family.**

How to Clean Fruits and Vegetables from Eggs and Larvae of Parasites

As discussed above, fruits, vegetables and berries can carry parasites and their eggs. The question becomes, "What can I do about it?"

Fruits and Vegetables

Fruits and vegetables should be washed with a special brush under running water. You can purchase special brushes, and fruits and vegetables rinses not containing harmful additives in health stores.

You can also use salt and lemon juice to wash fruits and vegetables. Mix one tablespoon of salt, one tablespoon of lemon juice, and one quart of water, pour the mixture over fruits or vegetables and let stand for 5-10 minutes.

Then thoroughly rinse 3-5 times in running water. Running water, if it's not filtered, also contains "uneatable" substances. Therefore dry your fruits and vegetables so the water can evaporate. Store vegetables in the refrigerator in boxes or ventilated plastic bags. There they can remain fresh for a few days to a few weeks. When you are getting ready to use them check their condition one more time. It's possible that you will have to cut some pieces out.

Berries

Be gentler when you clean strawberries, blueberries, raspberries, etc. You may use the same solution without the brush. Berries do not keep long even in the refrigerator, so try to eat them sooner than other fruits and vegetables.

Greens

- Separate greens from roots and other inedible parts.
- Rinse each plant under tap water and place in a large bowl.
- Pour in the bowl enough water that greens float on top.
- Add rinsing solution.
- Mix and shake the greens in the solution with your hands.
- Take out the greens and put them in a different container.
- Pour the water out of the bowl where you washed the greens. Rinse the bowl thoroughly. Rinse your hands of the rinsing solution.
- Pour clean water into the bowl and put the greens into the water.
- Once again move and shake the greens with your hands.
- Pour off the used water and add clean water and repeat the rinsing one more time.
- Repeat this **whole** process 3-5 times.
- Then the greens should be dried and consumed, or stored in the refrigerator in glass jars or plastic bags.

Your kitchen counter should be clean so that clean vegetables would not mix with unclean vegetables. Kitchen appliances such as juicers, blenders, food processors should also be thoroughly washed. Otherwise from technology that brings you health these could turn into sources of infection.

To kill parasites and their eggs in meat and fish products you have to thoroughly wash and then cook until completely ready. A way to get rid of fungus and parasite eggs in grain, nuts, seeds and beans is described in my book, *Deep Internal Body Cleansing*.

Diet and Parasites

Those who have candida probably notice that after they eat anything sweet they quickly feel gassy and bloated. Some even get irritations on their skin, allergies and other maladies.

These symptoms are big clues that something in our diet is activating the development of parasites. The thing to do is to stop activating them.

Products, which activate "sleeping" parasites and increase their numbers, include sweets of all kinds and also simple carbohydrates. That's why your diet should limit even the amount of sweet fruits and fruit juices. You can actually exclude those for some time, although, when making juices you can combine them in such a way as not to make them sweet, adding lemon juice, lime juice, celery, mustard greens etc.

Products, which limit activities of parasites and kill them, include **garlic, onion, pumpkinseed, lemon, cabbage, cranberries and cranberry juice, melon and its juice (use on an empty stomach).**

Small potatoes work well against small parasites. Pumpkinseed oil kills Trichomonas, candida, chlamydia and other parasites. Arrange your diet so that every meal includes one two or more components aimed at killing parasites. For example add lemon or cranberry juice to fruit juice. Cranberries can be added to protein shakes. You can add pumpkinseed oil to vegetable juices. Always mix fresh onions into your salads and garlic in your grains etc.

Fasting Against Parasites

Fasting takes away food from parasites (if the colon is cleansed beforehand). Fasting to eliminate parasites should be done on water with fresh onion juice (one teaspoon of onion juice to a cup of fresh water) or with cranberry juice (one teaspoon of cranberry juice to a cup of fresh water) or lemon juice (one to two teaspoons of lemon juice to one cup of fresh water). Preventive fasting should last one to three days every month. You can also do a one-day fast weekly.

Fasting without water, **dry fasting**, takes away not only food but also water from parasites. This is a difficult fast but overweight people with excess of water in their bodies can easily manage it. Dry fasting can be done one to two times a month for 24-36 hours.

Conclusion: The goal of all cleansing procedures described in this book is the battle with toxicity and parasites. Parasite infestation is a continuous process, and only a clean and healthy body can prevent their reproduction and transformation into disease. Therefore support the clean internal ecology of your body and fight against parasites as regularly as you brush your teeth, take a shower, etc.

Internal and external hygiene and responsibility for your health should become a part of the Daily Program of Your Life.

Remember, parasites need us. We do not need parasites. Whether or not you get rid of these unwelcome intruders is up to you. They take you very seriously. You should do no less with them.

The Next Book

To get the best results in the healing process, it is not enough to find a skilled teacher who can guide you along the path. It is also very important that the student be **open-minded** to new information and **ready to work.**

A Healthy Diet gives to the system not only nutrients but also help to clean and heal the body. To make your diet healthy, you need to learn

- Principles of Healthy Eating.
- Food Combining.
- When Is the Best Time for Digestion.
- How Much Food You Can Eat.
- What You Can Do to Improve Digestion.
- What You Can Eat on a Healing and Preventive Diet.
- Diet on a Daily Basis.
- Diet on Celebrations and for the Soul.
- Simple, Healthy Recipes of Living Foods and Spare Cooking.
- And Much More. . . .

People who want to lose weight will find in *Healing through Cleansing Diet, Book 4,* four simple programs for losing weight. These weight loss programs will help them lose not only weight but also their health disorders, while gaining enhanced health which looks and feels younger.

More Testimonials

"I Had Only Six Months to Live"
(Healing of Serious Kidney Disease in Two Weeks)

I had nephritis (kidney disease) for 14 years. In Russia the doctors didn't find out what exactly it was and how to treat it, but my kidneys were hurting so much with sharp, tingling pains. I came to America a couple of years ago still suffering with this disease.

One day several months ago both of my legs swelled up, and I went to the Emergency Room (ER). The ER doctor told me that he could not help me. My blood pressure started to fluctuate, rising and falling because of my nephritis, and I had headaches and dizziness.

I decided to go to the regular (traditional) doctor suggested by my insurance company, in this case a doctor of internal medicine. He did some testing and sent me to a urologist (doctor specializing in urinary problems). This second doctor looked at my lab test results (blood work, urinalysis), and after finding out my age, did some calculations that he said indicated that my kidneys worked only a 15% capacity. The urologist gave me one medicine for the swelling and another for killing infection. My swelling disappeared, but I still had a headache.

After one week, I came back again to the doctor and he gave me new medication for everything: kidney, blood pressure, and infection all in the same pill. I came home, took it, and begin to feel worse. I felt nausea, dizziness, headache, heart pain and palpitation. At the next appointment the doctor said he wanted me to do a kidney biopsy. I refused it. He also recommended that I have a kidney transplant, adding that I would have to find a good donor. He scared me and my family to death saying that I probably had only six months to live, that I would get so weak that I will not be able to function, and my family will have to take care of me till the day I die. The doctor said that he could not guarantee that a transplant could help and be successful. He said that after this surgery I would have to stay in bed for six months. When I came home, I stopped all medication because they didn't help, and I started to think about suicide. I wanted to find poison and die quietly without interrupting the life of my family.

After one week my daughter reminded me about Dr. Koyfman, who is well-known in the Russian community as an alternative health-care practitioner. We made an appointment, and I came to this office for consultation. Dr. Koyfman strongly recommended a special diet (no salt, no spice, no fermented food, no bread, no sugar, no meat, no sweets). He said that in order to get the results I needed I would have to follow his suggestions very strictly.

I was very committed to doing it because I wanted to survive. I didn't have any choice. I decided to follow every single thing that I needed to do. I made many changes all at the same time: doing special kidney massage and colon cleansing three times a week in the office, completely changing diet at home, drinking juices, eating fresh salads, cooking grains and soups sometimes adding olive oil only as a seasoning, doing special lower back light exercises and special light morning gymnastics, doing dry brush skin massage, jumping on the rebounder 10-15 minutes every day, walking outside for 30 minutes every day.

Before I came here I felt like a very old lady. I felt very weak, without energy, etc. Everything was very difficult to do. When I first came to the Center I could not even touch the kidney area, and the special kidney massage was very painful, but I was very committed to carrying through.

After two weeks, I started to feel better. My pain disappeared, and the massage is not painful anymore. I no longer use the back brace which was warming and supporting my lower back, and my colon functions normally now. I feel good, light, and young again. My swelling or edema has completely disappeared. The dark blue ring between and under my eyes disappeared. My ability to work and my energy level have increased. I can tell that I feel so much better without any medication or surgery, simply and naturally, and in only two weeks.

I wonder why the doctors don't seem to know about it. It seems strange because the first rule of medicine is to do no harm.

- *Mazol Yadgarova, 40 years old.* Atlanta, GA

"I Was Having a Lot of Pain"

I have been a client and patient of Dr. Koyfman's for approximately three years. I came to the Center after I was diagnosed with rheumatoid arthritis.

Before I came to Dr. Koyfman, I was having a lot of pain all over my body. I prayed and asked God for guidance on the path I should take to receive my healing. I believe God directed me to the Koyfman Center for Health and Rejuvenation because I wanted my health restored through natural methods.

I began a series of colonics and immediately started to feel better physically, but I knew that in order to totally restore my health, I was going to have to continue with deeper cleansing to remove all the toxins stored up in my body over the years.

I have had at least five liver cleanses, three joint cleanses, kidney, stomach, and small intestine cleanses, and along with the other natural methods used by the Center, including fasting, my overall health and quality of life have greatly improved.

I no longer have pain all over my body, my energy is better and my immune system is stronger.

Some of the other benefits I have received as a result of all the care from the Koyfmans is the ability to maintain a proper weight level and a healthier, thicker head of hair with natural curl restored, smoother skin and a tremendous wealth of knowledge on how to better take care of my physical body, an education in this area which is priceless!

In the world we live in today that is so environmentally toxic, I believe we must strive to improve our overall lifestyle through continuous detoxification methods such as the ones utilized at the Koyfman Whole Body Cleansing. In addition we must change to a healthy vegetarian diet, along with exercise and drinking sufficient amounts daily of pure water.

Dr. & Mrs. Koyfman are compassionate and caring health providers who can show you the way to achieve a better overall quality of life. I am a living testimony to this fact, and I am very grateful to the Koyfmans for helping me to continue to achieve my long-term goals for excellent health.

—*Hope Pitzer, Atlanta GA.*

"Thank God I Got Seriously Ill"

Believe it or not I am very thankful I became very, very ill [months at home in bed, doctor suggested surgery]. I am thankful for two reasons; 1) it forced me to take my health very seriously in a very big way, and 2) I met Dr. Koyfman. These two things in combination have made me healthier and more energetic than I can ever remember being. [Blood test before cell cleansing was abnormal, after cell cleansing, normal].

The Koyfman Whole Body Cleansing is a remarkable place. In addition to restoring health to an unhealthy body in a gentle way, the Center provides information and guidance to maintain a healthy body. There is no extra charge for the guidance and valuable information. Its just part of Dr. Koyfman's underlying belief that the Center's purpose is to help people stay healthy by keeping all the things that get you sick outside of your body. If any of those things get inside your body, the Koyfman Center will remove them. This is something conventional medicine cannot do.

Dr. Koyfman is a remarkable man. He has studied health in many countries and has earned many degrees. He has written many books. He started studying health before it was fashionable or popular. He was learning long before there were organic vegetable departments at the supermarket and he was learning before *Alternative Medicine* magazine was on the newsstand. But the most remarkable thing about Dr. Koyfman is his genuine desire to help. He really wants to help you get your health back, and then he really wants to help you maintain it. This is the thing that impressed me the most.

If I had only been slightly ill, rather than very ill, I probably would not have followed Dr. Koyfman's directives as close as possible. But since my illness was so serious I listened to every word. Thank God I did. Things happened just as Dr. Koyfman knew they would. My health recovered exactly as Dr. Koyfman told me it would happen, and if you follow Dr. Koyfman's directions precisely, he can restore your health too.

—*Steven Wenig, Atlanta, GA*

Unique Method of Colon Rejuvenation, 95 pages; $12.

Our bodies need constant help eliminating toxic substances which enter the system every day. Daily practice of the rising and restroom exercises described in this book strengthens colon muscles so that, with time, elimination will accompany each meal and eject more toxins than are retained. Also included are principles and recipes for healthy eating, raw meals, and safe cooking technology.

Eight Steps to Total Body Cleansing and Perfect Health, 214 pages; $20.

You will find here how to prepare for cleansing and what to expect during Deep Internal Body Cleansing. You will want to know what to do if you feel any discomfort during the cleansing. This book explains how we perform Deep Internal Body Cleansing at the Center. Also, you will discover here what to eat after the cleansing in order to maintain your success and your new lifestyle.

Deep Internal Body Cleansing, 172 pages. $15 plus shipping and handling.

If you search for healing and real health, then here you will find answers to your questions Here is information about toxicity and the immune system, healthy eating and eliminating parasites. Here are answers to help you resist hurtful cravings and negative emotions. You really can get health and gain energy through cleansing your body.

Healing Through Cleansing - Book 1, 114 pages; $12.

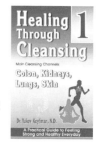

Every day, toxic substances enter our bodies from the various chemical and biological contaminants in our environment. Additionally, toxins form within us due to poor dietary habits, stress, aging, and harmful bacteria that populate our bodies. Our excretory organs can't cope with such a large amount of work and need constant, conscious support. How can you help your main excretory organs become free of toxins, bacteria, and infections? You will find the answers in the pages of this and subsequent books in this Koyfman Series.

Healing Through Cleansing - Book 2, 101 pages; $12.

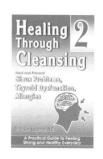

In many ways our health depends on the health of organs located in the head and neck regions: the brain, thyroid gland, eyes, salivary glands, ears, nose and sinuses, throat, tongue, teeth and gums. The contemporary American diet usually includes a large number of mucus-forming foods that result in the generation of mucus throughout the body. Excess mucus settles throughout the body, especially in the head and neck organs, giving rise to a number of ailments in these organs.

Healing Through Cleansing Diet - Book 4, 110 pages; $12.

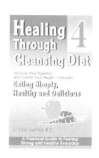

"To get the best results in the healing process, it is not enough to find a skilled teacher who can guide you along the path. It is also very important that the student be open-minded to new information and ready to work," says Dr. Yakov Koyfman, N.D. A healthy diet gives to the system not only nutrients but also help to clean and heal the body. To make your diet healthy, you need to learn the things in this book.